WOMEN AND HEART DISEASE

WOMEN and HEART DISEASE

EDWARD B. DIETHRICH, M.D.,
and
CAROL COHAN

BALLANTINE BOOKS · NEW YORK

To the women with heart disease whose diagnosis, treatment, and understanding made this book possible

—EBD

To the women whose lives have helped to define my own:
to Lena and to Lynn,
to Dina and to Debra,
to Janie,
and, most of all, to Bea, my mom

—CC

Copyright © 1992 by Edward B. Diethrich, M.D., and Carol Cohan
Afterword copyright © 1994 by Carol Cohan

All rights reserved under International and Pan-American Copyright Conventions. Published in the United States by Ballantine Books, a division of Random House, Inc., New York, and simultaneously in Canada by Random House of Canada Limited, Toronto.

This edition published by arrangement with Times Books, a division of Random House, Inc.

Library of Congress Catalog Card Number: 93-90474

ISBN: 0-345-38620-5

Cover design by Susan Grube

Manufactured in the United States of America

First Ballantine Books Edition: February 1994

10 9 8 7 6 5 4 3

ACKNOWLEDGMENTS

Like many books, this one began serendipitously. Ted Diethrich recognized the importance of a book on heart disease in women. Cassie Hill, director of public relations at the Arizona Heart Institute, came upon and liked a two-part magazine series I had written on the subject and brought the two of us together. Separately, my long-time and very dear friend Edna Povich brought me together with Gail Ross, Ted's and my agent. Gail's encouragement and enthusiasm were instrumental in developing this project. The first thanks belong to Cassie Hill, Edna Povich, and Gail Ross, who were indirectly responsible for the birth of this book.

This project is the product of partnership in the very best sense of the word: the merger of the two authors' respective talents and ideas into a single voice. I am indebted to my co-author for his collegiality, his availability, his flexibility, and his eagerness to facilitate the completion of this book in every way possible.

It went from preliminary research to finished manuscript in less than nine months. This feat required simultaneous researching, writing, revising, and constant updating as new data emerged. It never could have been accomplished without the expert, efficient, enthusiastic assistance of the professionals at the Arizona Heart Institute. Above all, I am indebted to Dr. Mary Grace Warner, clinical cardiologist, and Becky Bowman, director of research and editorial services.

Becky was my librarian and consultant. She ran literary searches, supplied me with reference materials as quickly as I requested them, faxed me new studies hot off the press, and helped me review statistical analyses and prepare the drug appendix. She also read early drafts of the manuscript, made valuable suggestions for revision, and was always available to kick around ideas.

Mary Grace embraced me as her shadow, and I trailed after her as she treated patients, reviewed their tests, and spoke with them about her findings. She devoted hours to giving me a thorough grounding in cardiology, and she reviewed the entire manuscript, answered endless questions, and served as an ongoing resource.

I am also grateful to the other physicians at the Arizona Heart Institute who permitted me to watch them work and who generously offered me their time, attention, and expertise: Michael Gordon, Richard Heuser, Sam Kinard, David Nelson, and L. Kent Smith. Also to the allied professionals who worked with me—Pat Arnold; David Hall, Ph.D.; Judy Milas, M.A., R.D.; Jayne Newmark, M.S., R.D.; Dana Riedel; Sterling Seaboch PA-C—and to the nurses and technicians who facilitated my research: Maureen Breading, R.N.; Sue Carroll, R.N.; Joyce Dunshee, R.N.; Brenda Nolan; and Eddie Trayler, R.N.

AHI's dedicated support staff also deserve abundant thanks. Margo Day, supervisor of transcriptions, and her department—Bonita Baker, Beth Garrish, and Judy Katz—spent many tedious hours transcribing interview tapes for me. The principals in Visual Arts Services—Spencer Phippen, Richard Williams, Chris Wooley, and their intern Judy Barr—were involved with this project from the outset and deserve credit for the illustrations that accompany this text. Ted Diethrich's office staff—Carol Mesquita, Bet LeVander, and especially Ginny Ziegler—coordinated my schedule and took good care of me during my research stints in Phoenix. Over the ensuing months, they promptly and cheerfully filled numerous requests for me long distance and played an important part in assuring that this project moved along in a timely fashion. I also appreciate the assistance of Susan Brada, Mary Facundus, Liz Hendricks, June McArdle, Faith McNeely, and Dorothy Seidman.

Many others, in addition to the staff at Arizona Heart Institute, made important contributions to this work, and I am indebted to all of them. Dr. Susan Light was an ongoing source of help and inspiration. So were Dr. Linda Tetrault and Dr. Pepi Granat. Betsy Singer, Ann Thomas, and especially Diane Stryar opened the doors of the National Institutes of Health to me. Debra Cohan, Dina Cohan, Dr. Bernard Cohen, Vicki Cohen, Andrea Fisch, Bess Marder, and Catherine Tuerk read early versions of some chapters. Dr. David Blumenthal and Dr. Charles Kalstone reviewed parts of the text and gave me valuable guidance.

And I am grateful to the scores of patients who bared their hearts to me. Julie Procich, founder of the national support group for young adults with heart disease, not only shared her own story but arranged for me to visit the Chicago chapter of Young Hearts and talk with their members. Subsequently, she answered more questions and orchestrated additional interviews. Julie, ever cheerful, ever positive, couldn't do enough. Neither could Pat Taylor, who first made Ted Diethrich aware of the seriousness of heart disease in women. Thank you to these two women for their important contributions to this project and for permitting their names to appear in print. Scores of other patients, whose stories appear under disguised identities, were equally helpful and candid. They enriched this book by allowing me to probe their most intimate experiences and feelings.

In the final stages of this work, the staff at Random House played an increasingly important role. I appreciate the contributions of Peter Smith as well as those of Nancy Inglis, Robbin Schiff, Martha Schwartz, and Naomi Osnos. I am particularly grateful to our editor, Betsy Rapoport. She is a tough taskmaster with keen instincts and a sharp eye. This text improved with every suggestion she made.

Most of all, I am thankful for the unfaltering understanding and tireless support of my family, especially my husband, Phil Glatstein. He read and reread every word of every draft, helped me refine my ideas, and articulate my thoughts. As always, he was a resilient sounding board and a brilliant devil's advocate. He was at once my severest critic and my most adoring fan. Both this book and I are blessed to have him on our team.

Carol Cohan
Miami, Florida

CONTENTS

INTRODUCTION

A fateful error occurred in medical research nearly half a century ago, and women have been paying for it ever since. At the time, the most ambitious and respected study of heart disease ever launched concluded that women were immune to it. Consequently, medical science turned its efforts to halting premature heart attacks in men. The American Heart Association entreated women to take care of their fathers, brothers, and husbands. A myth was born, and it lived for more than thirty years.

As the error came to light, the National Institutes of Health tried to remedy the blunder with their publication *The Healthy Heart Handbook for Women*. The American Heart Association began to boost awareness of "the silent epidemic" of heart disease in women. Newspapers, magazines, and television networks ran features on the subject. But the myth endures. Most Americans still don't know that women are vulnerable.

Ask anyone what the number-one killer of American women is, and chances are good that the answer will be breast cancer. In fact, breast cancer kills 44,000 American women every year. Heart disease kills over 500,000! The truth is: Heart disease is the number-one cause of death in women, just as it is in men. More shocking still, this development is not new; it's awareness of it that's new.

The good news is that, thanks to more healthful living and improved medical care, heart disease has been killing fewer people—men and women—in recent years than it did in the past. But because women have been excluded for so long from so many major medical studies of heart disease, we have a huge gap in our understanding of diagnosis and treatment.

Although much of the medical community is just waking up to the truth about heart disease in women, a young Long Island woman forced us at the Arizona Heart Institute to reckon with reality years ago. We had treated many women before her, but thirty-eight-year-old Pat Taylor captured our attention. Her case was striking because she was so young and because her disease was so profound that it required unconventional treatment. By 1980, Pat had had two heart attacks and two rounds of bypass surgery. When she traveled to Houston for go-round number three, her surgeon, one of this country's most-celebrated practitioners, threw up his hands in defeat and sent Pat home to die.

"I had two little boys," Pat recalled, "and there was no way I could give up the fight. I was desperate. I read about the Arizona Heart Institute and called them up."

The Arizona Heart Institute and Foundation, of which Ted Diethrich is director and chief surgeon, is the first freestanding outpatient center for the prevention, diagnosis, and treatment of heart and circulatory diseases. The institute evaluates new drugs, explores new ways to apply old knowledge, and pioneers new technologies, such as the use of lasers and other evolving alternatives to surgery. The challenge that Pat presented was right up our alley.

After evaluating Pat thoroughly, we agreed that surgery would not work for her. Pat was a frightening portrait of poor health. At five feet four inches, she weighed 153 pounds. Her cholesterol was inching its way toward 400. She was taking seven heart medications, yet she could not climb a flight of stairs without pain. If we couldn't operate, we had to come up with something else.

To decrease Pat's risk and protect her from further trouble, we changed her diet, improved her strength and stamina, gave her emotional support, and taught her how to manage stress. By penetrating every facet of her life, the program we devised for Pat began to turn her disability around.

Although Pat's heart was permanently scarred by disease, the program enabled her to compensate. In the eight weeks she spent at the institute in Phoenix, she lost sixteen pounds. In the supervised environment of cardiac rehabilitation, she lifted weights and did sit-ups, pedaled a bike, climbed stairs, and hiked up hills. Along the way, she developed enough stamina to raise her peak pulse to an impressive 158 without straining her heart. When she went back to Long Island, she took a personal prescription for sustaining the program. In the ensuing months, she lost an additional twenty-nine pounds and brought her blood pressure, cholesterol, triglycerides, and blood sugar into line. She eliminated her medications one by one and enjoyed complete freedom from pain. Twelve years later, despite periodic setbacks, Pat remains convinced that we were right in our initial prediction: If she continues to stay in charge of her heart's health, she is more likely to be hit by a bus at the age of eighty than to die of heart disease.

Working with Pat reminded us that we can't always fix the heart, and even when we can, the remedy is only temporary unless we also halt the process that caused the disease in the first place. In the ensuing years, we have customized her program hundreds of times, as we have done to meet the individual needs of men and women from throughout the country and help them accomplish similar goals.

In addition to inspiring this diet/exercise/stress-management plan, which came to be known as the Diethrich Program and which forms the basis of Chapter 10 in this book, Pat Taylor crystallized our awareness of the difficulties in diagnosing and treating women, and she helped to sharpen our strategies for confronting these dynamics head-on. In any given year at AHI, we see roughly seven women for every ten men. With this extensive involvement, we have personally experienced the discomfiting truths that medical research reports: Heart disease is particularly elusive and enigmatic in women. It is trickier to diagnose in women than in men, and we must sometimes implement innovative strategies to make reliable sense out of the test results we get. Women are also harder to treat, especially with surgery and other invasive techniques. So once heart disease asserts itself, women are more likely than men to suffer permanent disability or to die.

Because of these potential problems, prevention and prompt intervention are paramount. The sooner you define your risk and begin to reduce it, the better your chance of holding disease at bay. To help accomplish this, researchers at the Arizona Heart Institute and Foundation devised the Heart Test for Women, which you'll find in Chapter 3. This test, a statistically reliable written survey based on years of data, had its origin in a similar survey prepared by the AHI Foundation in 1981. Like its predecessor, which made its debut on ABC's 20/20 and was the focus of *Heart Test* (Cornerstone Library, 1981), the new test will help you assess your risk of heart disease depending on your age; family and personal history; whether you have diabetes; your smoking, eating, and exercise habits; and your levels of cholesterol, blood pressure, and stress. The new test also reflects the unique dynamics of heart disease in women that have come to light in recent years.

When you take this test and tabulate your score, you will know whether your personal risk of heart disease is low, medium, or high, so you will be in a strategic position to take preventive measures. If you already have heart disease, you will learn what you can do possibly to slow its progress, even if you've already had a heart attack or bypass surgery. If you have no signs of disease yet, maybe you can prevent it. And if you know you are at risk, you can arrange to get competent, comprehensive medical care.

This is easier said than done. Not only do we know less about heart disease in women than in men, but several recent studies confirm that women with heart disease face bias in their diagnosis and treatment. Their symptoms are more likely to be misinterpreted, overlooked, or dismissed as psychosomatic. Consequently, some women are never properly diagnosed and die unnecessarily. Others are diagnosed so late in the game that the potential benefits of treatment are compromised. (We'll discuss the roots of that bias in Chapter 1.) Where the commodity is health care, the price of ignorance and bias can be enormous. And sad to say, it is a price that many women with heart disease have had to pay.

Ethel Davis is a prime example. When she first developed chest pain, she went to her doctor, who did everything wrong. He did not say, "This could be serious. We must find out what is causing your pain." He did not prescribe an appropriate workup. He did not acknowledge that diagnosing and treating heart disease in women is particularly puzzling. He did not admit the limits of his own ability. And he did not refer Ethel to a specialist.

Meanwhile, weeks stretched into months and then into years. As the pain gradually grew worse, Ethel's physician looked for a disease of the immune system and ruled it out. He looked for gallbladder disease and ruled it out. He looked for hiatal hernia and ruled it out. He never really considered heart disease until Ethel tried to hike the hills in San Francisco and pain stopped her short.

Before Ethel's saga ended, this same physician, who had side-stepped a methodical cardiac workup for so long, would railroad Ethel into a delicate and invasive cardiac catheterization at a hospital unequipped to manage the complications that could ensue. He would whisk her from cardiac catheterization into an inadvisable and ill-fated balloon angioplasty, which, in turn, catapulted her into emergency bypass surgery fraught with complications and a checkered recovery. Manipulated by her physician's charm and poor judgment from the outset, she never even got a second opinion.

The purpose of this book is to save you from Ethel's fate by giving you the kind of background you need to ask the right questions and form an effective partnership with a good doctor. Considering the breadth and complexity of cardiology, this is a tall order. To accomplish it we tapped the talents of several key people with different disciplines and perspectives at Arizona Heart Institute, chief among them Mary Grace Warner, M.D., a clinical cardiologist and echocardiography specialist with extensive experience in diagnosing and treating women. Formerly on the cardiology faculty at Michigan State University, Dr. Warner worked closely on this project to assure that the information presented in the coming chapters reflects the most current research and sophisticated thinking. Former AHI director of nutritional services Jayne Newmark and her successor, Judy Milas, contributed their talents to this project. So did L. Kent Smith, M.D., M.P.H., director of cardiac rehabilitation services; David Hall, Ph.D., director of psychological services; Becky Bowman, medical editor and director of scientific information services, and Pat Arnold, science writer.

This book cannot and must not replace hands-on medical care or the specific advice of your doctor. Use it instead to help you ask the right questions, make the right choices, question suspicious practices or oversights, and protect your rights as a patient. Use it, too, as a guide to prevention: to treating your body more kindly and to protecting your life.

WOMEN AND HEART DISEASE

CHAPTER 1

The Truth About Heart Disease in Women

Early in December 1990, sixty-two-year-old Betty Richards felt a deep, dull pain spread across her chest, down her left arm, and up into her jaw. She went immediately to a local emergency clinic, where the physician concluded she was suffering from anxiety. He advised her to take it easy and sent her home. Betty felt the pain twice more. Each time she went back to the clinic. Each time the doctor said she was suffering from anxiety and sent her home. And then, just before Christmas, Betty died. Her autopsy confirmed the cause of her death: massive heart attack.

Betty should not have died this way. Obviously, her physician never considered that she might be suffering from heart disease, and he failed to take the necessary steps to protect her life. Worse, Betty is not unusual. Time and again women have reported that their physicians do not take their complaints seriously. That when they suffer from chest pain their physicians give them Valium, but when their husbands experience identical symptoms, the same physicians order cardiac workups. That even when women have confirmed heart disease and the test results to prove it, doctors sometimes refuse to accept the diagnosis.

The sad truth is that many American physicians—in fact, most American people—hold on to the delusion that heart disease is reserved for men. All the while, a silent epidemic rages through the female population.

AN EQUAL-OPPORTUNITY KILLER

More than ten million women have some cardiovascular problem. By age forty-five, heart disease affects one woman in nine. By age sixty-five, that ratio becomes one in three. And although heart disease is more prevalent among men, it is more deadly for women. Compared to a man, a woman who suffers a heart attack is more like to die. If she survives, she is more vulnerable to a second attack and chronic, disabling chest pain. If she has bypass surgery or balloon angioplasty, she is less likely to survive. And if she does, she is less likely to recover fully.

Heart attacks kill 520,000 people every year, and nearly half of them —247,000—are women. Add strokes, usually caused by blockages in the arteries that lead to the brain, and the female death count increases by 90,000. Deaths from all cardiovascular diseases combined claim half a million women's lives every year, more than double the 220,000 deaths from all kinds of cancer. As the American Heart Association wryly observes, heart disease is an equal-opportunity killer.

The reality is scandalous: Physicians are overlooking the primary cause of death in half the American population. The Surgeon General of the United States is a woman. The director of the National Institutes of Health is a woman. Nearly one in five practicing physicians is a woman. And better than one medical student in three is a woman. Yet women continue to be turned away from their physicians' offices with a pat on the head and a patronizing nod.

THE HISTORY OF SEXISM IN MEDICINE

Contemporary cardiac care is just one example of discriminatory medical practice. Penetrating every facet of the medical profession, this bias is deeply rooted in the centuries-old stereotype that women are weak and complaining while men are strong and stoic. Two hundred years ago, it was commonly believed that intellect and economic success were gifts bestowed by virtue of male gender, specifically the genitals, while physical frailty and emotional fragility were

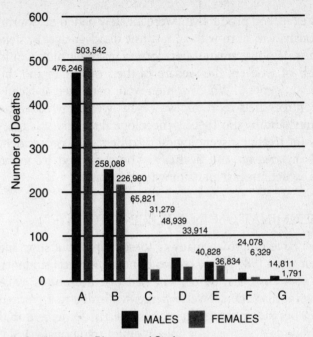

Leading Causes of Death in the United States in 1988

A Cardiovascular Disease and Stroke
B Cancer
C Accidents
D Chronic Obstructive Pulmonary Disease
E Pneumonia and Influenza
F Suicide
G AIDS

Source: National Center for Health Statistics and the American Heart Association.

caused by women's reproductive organs. These beliefs found their way into earliest medical practice. In 1872, for example, Dr. Augustus Kinsley Gardner wrote that "the concentrated powers of man's perfected being" were found in his sperm, "the purest extract of the blood . . . *totus homo semen est.*" In 1835, an article in the *Boston Medical and Surgical Journal* warned that intemperate discharge of sperm could drain the energies of the system. Men feared that frequent ejaculation would weaken their seed and produce runts, feeble infants, and girls. Worse, wasted sperm meant lost intellectual energy and productive capability. Drained of their essence, men would diminish their capacity to earn money, win wars, and otherwise shape the destiny of mankind.

If a male's intellect and productivity were innately tied to his sperm, a female, obviously, was born with an intrinsic disadvantage. By definition, women were not as smart. Men worried that education would harm the health of women, the welfare of their offspring, and the future of society in general. While women were perceived as having superior self-control, their reproductive organs were viewed as the source of insanity, and by the 1860s, gynecological surgery was practiced expressly for treating psychological disorders. It is no accident that the words *hysterectomy* and *hysteria* are both derived from the Greek *hysterikos*, which means "pertaining to the womb."

DISCRIMINATION IN MEDICINE TODAY

As a society, we have outgrown many of these beliefs, but shocking remnants remain. In a 1984 survey of two hundred medical students, three-quarters of them male, 34 percent said that hormones make women less logical than men. Twelve percent affirmed that women are less creative because of their hormones. Nearly 20 percent said that a genetic rationale justifies the jobs women traditionally hold. And better than half believed that women seek medical attention more than men because women are anxious about their bodies.

If these students didn't bring their bias to medical school with them, they would have been taught it once they got there. In the 1970s, when today's fortysomething physicians were students, the *New England Journal of Medicine* took a stand and condemned lecturers for traditionally referring to patients as "he" except in the context of psychological disorders, which they customarily discussed in terms of "she." In the intervening years, little has changed. In 1991, students at Stanford Medical School complained that professors lecture as though they were speaking only to men. Although women make up half the class, one professor discussing uterine contractions allegedly said, "You may never feel any of this, but your wife will." Another professor is accused of peppering his lectures with slides of *Playboy* centerfolds, and still another was brought up on formal charges of misconduct, having been accused of denying a student a teaching assistantship because she refused him sexual favors. Stanford dean David Korn, M.D., accepted the blame. "There is a whole range of stereotypic behavior that arises from a male-dominated culture. It would be nonsense to say sexism doesn't exist."

In fact, the medical profession is a bastion of sexism. Although the government's two top medical posts are held by women and the percentage of women in medical school rose from 9 percent in 1970 to 37 percent in 1990, only 20 percent of medical school teachers nationwide are women, and they occupy the lower ranks. Only 10 percent of full professors are women and only 4 percent are department heads. There are no female deans of medical schools, and only four female assistant deans. In its 144-year history, the American Medical Association has never had a woman as chief executive officer.

A survey of female practitioners in Massachusetts revealed that 54 percent encountered some form of sex discrimination in their professional lives. Twenty-seven percent reported sexual harassment, while 55 percent were bothered by milder forms of unwanted sexual attention. Sharyn Lenhart, M.D., and her co-authors of this survey, published in the July/August 1991 issue of the *Journal of the American Medical Women's Association*, observed, "We no longer pound on the entry gates —instead, we bump against glass ceilings that keep us from reaching our full potential for leadership and job satisfaction."

Discrimination is further reflected in earnings. According to a report released by the Feminist Majority Foundation and the American Medical Women's Association in September 1991, female physicians earned just 63.2 cents for each dollar a male physician earned in 1982, and in 1988 that number was down to 62.8 cents. American Medical Association figures confirm the trend. In 1987, female doctors with up to four years' experience earned $74,000, compared to the $110,600 earned by male doctors with comparable experience. Women with ten to twenty years' experience made $99,400, compared to $158,800 for men.

When this sexism is translated into patient care, women's complaints are treated as trivial while men's are presumed to be significant. Perhaps this practice grows out of the tendency for women to seek medical attention for minor complaints while men are more inclined to wait for a crisis. Regardless of why, the problem is real. More than once the *New England Journal of Medicine* has criticized medical practitioners for portraying women as hysterical patients and treating them in an "inadequate" and "derisory" way. Similarly, a study published in the *Journal of the American Medical Association* concluded that physicians presume illness to be more serious if the patient is male. Interestingly, the authors of this research had hoped to prove just the opposite. Tired of hearing about discrimination against women, they selected a prestigious group of family practitioners in California and audited the medical records of over one hundred male and female patients with identical complaints, among them fatigue, dizziness, and chest pain. To the researchers' surprise and chagrin, they found the men consistently received more extensive workups than the women.

On a larger scale, these trends reflect a pervasive practice of keeping women from thorough testing and aggressive treatment for heart disease. Two studies published in July 1991 documented this bias, reporting that although women commonly experience angina, they do not receive testing as routinely as men. When they do undergo non-invasive tests and these tests suggest the existence of coronary heart disease, they are not uniformly referred for cardiac catheterization, which is prerequisite to any invasive treatment. This testing pattern proves that even though women are more disabled by angina than men, women receive aggressive treatment half as often.

One of the new studies to make this point looked at over two thousand patients with acknowledged coronary heart disease, 17 percent of them female, at 112 hospitals in the United States and Canada. The other study assessed over eighty thousand patients, almost half of them women, in Maryland and Massachusetts. Together this research reflects discriminatory practices of countless physicians in two nations. And in April 1992, four additional studies reaffirmed the trend.

Not every physician is guilty of discriminatory practice. Many, many women get prompt, definitive care for heart disease and other conditions. Yet medical discrimination against women is rampant enough for the American Medical Association to have officially condemned it in 1990. Noting that women are deprived of critical attention for lung cancer and kidney disease as well as aggressive management of heart disease, the Council on Judicial and Ethical Affairs observed. "Gender bias may not necessarily manifest itself as an overt discrimination based on sex. Rather, social attitudes, including stereotypes, prejudices, and other evaluations based on gender roles may play themselves out in a variety of ways." Taking care to stop short of direct accusation, the AMA advised practitioners to look inward, asserting, "The medical community cannot tolerate any discrepancy in the provision of care that is not based on appropriate biological or medical indications."

Thus, throughout its history, American medicine has been infused with a gender bias that persists today. In this environment of prejudice, the seminal research on heart disease took place.

Little was known about heart disease before the middle of the twentieth century. From the time of Hippocrates, physicians had noticed that older men were its primary targets. In later centuries, they observed that heart disease seemed to run in families and appeared tied to high blood pressure and fat-laden diets. But observations were casual and the theories behind them unsubstantiated by reliable statistics. As for meaningful understanding of the disease itself, autopsies had revealed that heart attacks occurred as the result of blockages in the coronary arteries. Period.

Meantime, the number of victims kept growing: 165 for every 100,000 Americans in 1900, 200 per 100,000 in 1920, and 250 per 100,000 in 1930. Observers, notably the brilliant Harvard cardiologist Paul Dudley White, reasoned that physicians could never hope to contain the epidemic unless they understood it more clearly. Who was at risk? What put them there? How did the condition assert itself?

The only way to answer questions like these was to enlist a population before they got sick and study everything about them that might be pertinent. The researchers would obtain data periodically over several decades and wait for disease to appear. In this posture of watchful waiting, the researchers hoped to identify underlying causes, trace valid trends, and thereby build a foundation of reliable, meaningful knowledge.

THE LEGACY OF FRAMINGHAM

For their laboratory, researchers chose Framingham, Massachusetts, a small town near Boston whose residents rarely moved away, and they selected just over 5,000 healthy people—2,282 men and 2,845 women, ranging in age from thirty to sixty-two. Every two years, beginning in 1948, the participants submitted to thorough examinations, blood tests, lung-capacity measurements, body-fat calibrations, and more. They answered questions about personality characteristics, emotional traits, and living habits. The investigators charted their illnesses and hospitalizations. And when they died, the researchers studied why. In the forty years since the study began, the researchers lost track of only 3 percent of the original group, a circumstance that lends the study extraordinary credence.

Framingham is the first—and remains the largest—ongoing study of heart disease to include women and men in virtually equal numbers. Because the study began with healthy volunteers, the researchers approached their discoveries without preconceived expectations. Because of its impeccable design, the Framingham Study, probably more than any other, has made a profoundly positive impact on cardiac health and health care.

The Framingham Study, for example, deserves credit for discovering that certain conditions provoke heart attacks, and that susceptibility increases as these conditions become more pronounced. Out of this insight came the expression "risk factors," the now-common phrase that refers to the ways that vulnerability to illness is affected by age, family history, smoking, cholesterol, blood pressure, hormones, blood sugar, weight, activity level, and stress.

Moreover, as Chapter 3 will discuss in depth, analyses out of Framingham highlighted some marked differences in the way risk factors work in women as compared to men. It documented, for example, that women with high blood pressure were three times as likely to suffer a heart attack as those with normal blood pressure, while the ratio in men was 2 to 1.

Paradoxically, however, the purity of this study's design—the very essence of its virtue—was also responsible for its great blunder. Without any preconceived ideas about what they might find (except, perhaps, the presumption that women tend to be hypochondriacal) and without any other study results against which to evaluate their own, the Framingham investigators were unwittingly lured into drawing false conclusions about heart disease in women.

Their first reports came out in the mid-fifties, several years before the development of coronary angiography, which permits the arteries of the heart to be seen. At the time, chest pain was considered significant only if it resulted in a heart attack. During those first six years, ninety-eight Framingham participants had heart attacks. Eighty-one of them were men. Aside from seventeen women who suffered heart attacks, forty-four complained of chest pain that showed no signs of being life threatening. Thus, the researchers observed, heart disease afflicts men predominantly; even when women get it, the condition doesn't appear to be serious.

Without being able to view the coronary arteries, the researchers had no objective way to evaluate chest pain. And because the researchers were charting virgin territory, they had no way to know that the great majority of women in their study, then thirty-six to sixty-eight years old, were too young to have heart attacks. No one had yet discovered that women develop heart disease ten years after men and that heart attacks strike women another ten years down the road. Without this key information, the seeds of misconception began to germinate.

The next reports, issued in 1960, when the participants ranged in age from forty-two to seventy-four, appeared to support the initial presumption. After twelve years, 69 percent of affected women continued to experience intermittent chest pain, which the researchers had already determined was benign. In contrast, heart attacks struck 70 percent of the men without prior warning. Moreover, the men died at triple the rate of women. Since this observation paralleled national mortality statistics, the only corroborating data available, the researchers assumed their observations to be valid. However, the participants in the study were still too young to highlight the differences between heart disease in men and women. It would be years before the medical researchers would discover that unlike the disease in men, which tends to strike suddenly and acutely beginning when men are in their mid-forties, the disease in women sets in slowly. Characteristically, when women are in their fifties or sixties, they develop transient heart pain, which gradually gets worse before a heart attack strikes. Since this critical difference was yet unrecognized, the myth and its resulting complacency continued to grow.

The first two reports from Framingham appeared to confirm popular impressions: It was the men who were dramatically and prematurely dropping dead from heart disease—the thirty-five-year-old who perished on the tennis court, the forty-two-year-old who was fatally stricken while shoveling snow, the fifty-three-year-old who succumbed before he could pull his car off the highway. Moreover, in the 1950s and 1960s, when these data emerged, coronary heart disease seemed to be racing out of control in America. The trend begun earlier in the century accelerated. Heart attacks killed more and more people until 1963; while death rates from other diseases, including strokes, began to decline in 1950.

When mortality statistics plus the Framingham data suggested that the crisis targeted middle-aged men, the disease became synonymous with this population. Consequently, with few exceptions, notably the exhaustive Harvard Nurses Health Study, all subsequent heart disease research focused on men. For example, the Veterans Administration

Cooperative Study, one of the first and largest evaluations of coronary bypass surgery (686 men); the Multiple Risk Factor Intervention Trial, appropriately nicknamed "Mr. Fit," which assessed the merits of modifying cardiac risk factors (13,000 men); the oft-cited Physician's Health Study, which endorsed aspirin for preventing heart disease (22,000 men); the Harvard School of Public Health survey, which vindicated coffee as a cause of heart disease (over 45,000 men—and *not one woman*). Excluding women from research reinforced the misconception: Heart disease is a malady of men.

THE TRUTH EMERGES

The truth about heart diseases in women quietly began to appear in the mid-sixties, when a population study in Tecumseh, Michigan, similar to the Framingham project, revealed that women don't recover from heart attacks as well as men. Then, in 1982, Framingham's great error was exposed.

By 1982, coronary angiography, which captures X-ray images of the heart and its arteries, had become commonplace. That year, publication of the Coronary Artery Surgery Study, a review of over a thousand patients in several major medical centers, revealed that half the women referred for catheterization, compared to just 17 percent of men, did not have blocked arteries. Researchers knew that patients were referred for cardiac angiography if they complained of chest pain. Given this axiom, if half the women referred had clear arteries, something other than coronary artery disease had to be causing their pain. For the first time, researchers realized that all chest pain, especially in women, does not come from coronary artery disease.

This revelation blew away a major premise of the Framingham work and sent the researchers back to their calculators. Reevaluating their work, the investigators realized that they had erroneously presumed all chest pain to emanate from coronary artery disease, when, in fact, much of it did not. When they eliminated chest pain caused by other conditions and recalculated, they discovered the truth: Compared to men, fewer women develop coronary heart disease, they develop it later in life, and they develop it more gradually. But once the disease asserts itself, it is worse for women. It is more crippling, it is more deadly, and most frightening of all, it is more difficult to diagnose.

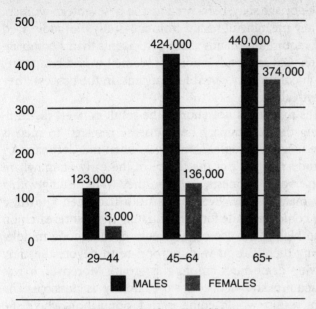

Estimated Annual Number of Americans, by Age and Sex, Experiencing Heart Attack

MALES   FEMALES

Source: Based on the Framingham Heart Study, 26-year follow-up.
Reproduced with permission from *1992 Heart and Stroke Facts*, 1991, p. 21. Copyright © American Heart Association, Dallas, Texas.

DISCRIMINATION PERSISTED

One would expect that revelations of this magnitude would shake up the medical community. But just the opposite happened. There were no headlines to alert practitioners or patients. There were no systematic revisions in medical school curricula, where heart disease was traditionally promulgated as a disease of men. And there was no attempt to close the research gap.

In fact, for almost another decade the National Institutes of Health intentionally and systematically continued to exclude women from one study after the next, despite congressional mandate to include them. Researchers claimed they could not study women of childbearing age, particularly if drugs were involved, because participants might become pregnant and then their babies would be jeopardized. Researchers further avoided women under fifty because their cycling hormones made analysis more difficult. And people over sixty-five, the age group comprising most female heart patients, were traditionally excluded because they were likely to have other illnesses or die from other causes, which would also complicate the research task.

Mostly, though, they were deterred by cost. Because one in five men has a heart attack by age sixty, compared to one in seventeen women, getting statistically meaningful results from any study of middle-aged women would require thousands more participants than a comparable study of men. Consequently studies of women would cost more, and the research community opted for bargains. In the process, they kept the old myth alive.

To be fair, this practice is not entirely the result of overt discrimination. Devoting the preliminary heart disease research to men is understandable, even justifiable. Until 1982, when the Coronary Artery Surgery Study pointed out the fallacy of the early Framingham conclusions, researchers honestly believed they were dealing with a predominantly male disease. Even if the truth had been known, a valid argument could be made for concentrating the first research on men. Given the high incidence of premature death among middle-aged men during the 1950s, it was appropriate to devote the early studies to slowing death rates among this group. Moreover, it was important to acquire knowledge as expeditiously as possible. The most expedient results would come from a population where the problem was concentrated and confounding variables were minimal —in other words, a population of middle-aged men.

Moreover, some responsibility for male-centered research lies with the women's liberation movement. The women's movement was gaining momentum just as the early studies on men were being designed, and feminist attitudes of the 1970s tacitly condoned the practice. As Bernadine Healy, M.D., director of the National Institutes of Health, told the Senate Labor and Human Resources Aging Subcommittee in April 1991, "For all its value, the women's liberation movement had one unfortunate side effect: an emphasis on 'sameness' in men and women. . . . With this backdrop, it is not surprising that biomedical research conducted these past twenty years has not focused on differences between men and women, but rather on women being just like men."

Finally, until research practices changed to include people over sixty-five, the female population most affected by heart disease could not be studied. Since heart disease in women is primarily a disease of older people and since this group was excluded from research, women were disproportionately excluded. Within the last ten years, the population of older people has exploded. With those over eighty-five comprising the fastest growing segment of the population, understanding the health and illness of aged men and women has become a priority. But it is a new priority, and it is unfair to evaluate the need for knowledge today based on the demographics of a decade ago.

What is disturbing is not that women were barred from early research but that they continue to be excluded from heart disease research even in recent years and that this practice conforms to a pervasive pattern of male-dominated research in one specialty after the next. As Dr. Healy wrote in a *New England Journal of Medicine* editorial, women have been "second-class and less than equal for most of recorded time and throughout most of the world. It may therefore be sad, but not surprising, that women have all too often been treated less than equally in social relations, political endeavors, business, education, research, and health care."

The truth is, researchers simply don't think in terms of women. Animal research conducted in the 1950s suggested that estrogen protected women from coronary heart disease, but the concept was not tested on women for decades. Instead, hormone therapy was tested on men, and when it caused them to develop blood clots, estrogen was presumed to promote heart disease in all people. To this day, some physicians still hold on to this mistaken belief.

Separate from logic, a research bias exists because most researchers are men. In nursing, parenthetically, where investigators, reviewers, and journal editors are predominately female, research has concentrated on female issues and involved female subjects, but nursing research has traditionally received less money than other specialties. Aside from nursing, there are few women researchers, reviewers, and administrators in high places, and female illnesses have traditionally gotten short shrift. There is no institute especially for obstetrics and gynecology at the NIH, and until now there has been little research on menopause, osteoporosis, ovarian cancer, or breast cancer. "I've had a theory that you fund what you fear," said Representative Pat Schroeder, co-chair of the Congressional Caucus for Women. "When you have a male-dominated group of researchers, they are more worried about prostate cancer than breast cancer."

Whether or not this theory is valid, the fact remains that medical research—on heart disease, on other diseases, on drugs, even on normal human growth and development—has consistently focused on middle-aged white men. For example, the National Institute on Aging has supported the Baltimore Longitudinal Study of Aging since 1958. Although the study began including women in 1978, its 1984 report, considered a definitive treatise on the phenomenon of aging, was based solely on male data. For another example, AIDS research has concentrated almost exclusively on men, even though approximately one in every ten HIV-positive persons is female and, by 1993, AIDS is projected to be among the top five causes of death for women under age forty-four. Data on men drives our understanding of psychological disorders and the development of cold remedies, even diet pills. Thus, when researchers made little attempt to close the knowledge gap once the truth about heart disease in women came out, their behavior followed a well-established pattern of disregard.

CHANGING THE PRACTICE

Gradually critics began to realize that a contradiction was driving the science community. On the one hand, researchers excluded women because the effects of their hormones made them too complex to study. On the other hand, researchers claimed women should be treated just like men. This contradiction underscored the reality that women and men are separate and distinct biological entities. Women have different patterns of disease and health and different responses to treatment.

By 1985, the U.S. Public Health Service Task Force on Women's Health Issues reported the information gap on the health needs of women, especially women of color, and mandated the NIH to include women and minorities in their studies and to analyze their results by gender. Accordingly, the NIH, which is part of the Public Health Service and the principal federal agency supporting medical research, established an advisory committee on women's health issues, to assure that the recommendations of the task force were fulfilled. In addition, in 1985 the NIH sponsored a conference on heart disease in older people and one in women in 1986. These two meetings outlined vast gaps in knowledge, and in October 1986, the NIH announced a new policy that encouraged independent researchers seeking NIH funds to include women in their studies. Tentative and indifferent, the policy did not require that women be included in research, and investigators employed directly by NIH were exempt. Although the policy was reiterated in January 1987, the NIH spent only 14 percent of its $7.6 billion research budget on women's health issues that year. In 1988, that proportion was down to 13.5 percent. By June 1989, the NIH still had not yet published clear and specific guidelines for implementing the new policy.

In December 1989, Representatives Pat Schroeder and Olympia Snow, co-chairs of the Congressional Caucus for Women, together with Henry Waxman, chairman of the House Subcommittee on Health and the Environment, requested an audit of NIH grants by Congress's inspection agency, the General Accounting Office (GAO). Specifically, the representatives wanted to know how the task force recommendations had changed NIH policy. When the GAO presented its findings to Congress the following June, it reported a sham.

The GAO found, for example, that NIH had ignored its new policy for three years. NIH first alerted its staff to the details of the policy in July 1989, and in the ensuing months, NIH staff continued to be confused and uncertain about it. Grant application reviewers did not begin to apply the policy until February 1990, and even then did not do so consistently. During the spring of 1990, an application for an all-male study of coronary artery disease won preliminary approval for funding on the rationale that the disease afflicts more men than women.

Those who plan the research projects and request funding learned about the policy last. Not until August 1990 did NIH specify how research should be designed to include women and minorities. Consequently, the GAO audit, which was filed the preceding June, reported that some 20 percent of proposals ignored gender entirely in their discussions of study populations. Where women had been included, study results were not analyzed by gender. In short, as of June 1990, little progress toward understanding the health needs of women had been made.

THE CONSEQUENCES OF DISCRIMINATION

Where heart disease is concerned, the consequences of this travesty have been astronomical. For starters, excluding women from research implicitly reinforced the notion that women are immune to heart disease and engendered a perilous ignorance among the general public. Countless women who had no idea they were susceptible have suffered heart attacks without knowing it. Sixty-eight-year-old Rose Mercer is one of them. For months, Rose had periodically experienced a heavy feeling in her chest, which she presumed was indigestion. It never lasted long, and she never gave it any thought. One evening, the sensation seemed a little stronger than usual, and Rose took some Maalox. Although the discomfort subsided slightly, it never quite went away. When she went to bed that night, she felt short of breath until she propped herself up on several pillows. The pain persisted for two days, and finally Rose went to the hospital. Because Rose did not recognize the heart attack as it was happening, she did not get to the hospital for emergency care, which often averts permanent damage. By the time she learned that she had heart disease, a considerable portion of her heart muscle was dead.

Rose's experience jibes with research that suggests women suffer permanent injury because they delay getting treatment. In a crisis where minutes matter, women get to the hospital on average three hours later than men, one study reported. It also revealed that, while women like Rose would have taken decisive action if they had realized what was happening, others don't know enough about heart attacks and emergency treatment to look after themselves. Heart attack symptoms can range from imperceptible to excruciating, and if women don't even know they are vulnerable, they cannot hope to identify symptoms that can be mystifying.

Worse, some physicians are also unaware, and, as the story at the very beginning of this chapter reveals, this ignorance sometimes costs patients their lives. More commonly, physicians miss the opportunity to identify women at risk and implement the preventive strategies that have worked so well for men.

Worst of all, the practice of excluding women from research has left an enormous gap in knowledge regarding diagnosis of heart disease in women. During the sixties, seventies, and eighties, technology revolutionized cardiac care. These were the decades when computers, ultrasound, and radioactive isotopes transformed diagnosis. During these decades, open-heart surgery matured and space-age treatments within the blood vessels themselves were born. All these developments were devised and evaluated mostly with men in mind. And just as the medical establishment finally recognized their oversights, researchers also began to discover that the differences between men and women are more profound than anyone had ever imagined.

This gap in knowledge has clearly taken a toll on women's well-being. As the Framingham researchers finally discovered, heart disease in women usually develops gradually, with some kind of warning before a major attack. It would seem, then, that with proper monitoring and testing, women could avert disaster. However, the primary warning sign—chest pain called angina, which signals insufficient blood flow to the heart from time to time—is frequently disguised and indiscernible in women. To compound this problem, women, much more than men, are vulnerable to an array of innocuous chest pains. Consequently, women and their physicians often fail to distinguish significant sensations from insignificant ones, and symptoms that should provoke concern are often overlooked.

If there were an inexpensive, noninvasive screening mechanism that was reliable in women, the problem would be less daunting. But diagnostic technologies, which have been developed for men, don't work as well for women. The only way to get a firm grip on the disease in women is by cardiac catheterization, a relatively safe but invasive procedure that costs upward of $5,000. Given the cost, a remote risk of heart attack or death, and the results of the 1982 Coronary Artery Surgery Study, which showed that half the women referred for catheterization had clear arteries, the test has yet to become accepted for routine evaluation in many institutions. Because researchers have not developed dependable screening tests for heart disease in women, many fail to get diagnosed in the early stages of illness, when treatment might hold greater promise.

If clinicians look for heart disease in their female patients and find it, research provides little guidance for aggressive treatment. There are no clinical trials on angioplasty in women, and in the few studies on bypass surgery in which women were included, the numbers are tiny and the conclusions grim. Although no study has ever clarified why, the available research consistently finds that women die or suffer serious complications twice as often as men. One study advised physicians recommending bypass for female patients to warn that surgery is risky and its benefits uncertain. Who could blame a clinician for shunning aggressive treatment for women on the basis of research like this?

Without a reliable body of research to guide them, many practitioners tread cautiously. If women get aggressive treatment at all, it is likely to take place under emergency conditions, when risks are always greater. The paucity of female-centered research has thus tied physicians' hands and indirectly fostered their discrimination against their female patients. As a result, once heart disease asserts itself, women are especially prone to early death or permanent disability.

The disadvantage that women have suffered is not unique to heart disease. Although one in ten women will someday develop breast cancer, only $17 million was spent on breast cancer research in 1989. With little attention to the medical conundrums of women, menopause has been the subject of scant research even though it directly affects heart disease, osteoporosis, and cancers of the breast and uterus. Consequently, although women live longer than men—seven years on average—they do so in poorer health. Two thirds of America's aging population are women who outlive their husbands and hobble into old age alone. Half of them will spend at least a year in a nursing home before they die because medical wisdom has found a way to extend their lives but not the means to prolong their independence.

The solution is not to build more nursing homes but to halt the onslaught of heart disease before it becomes crippling and to prevent the other disabilities of old age. Women might be stronger if physicians knew how to prevent the bone loss that leads to hip fractures, or if women were not 30 percent less likely than men to receive kidney transplants, or if vulnerable women were screened for lung cancer with the same vigor that men are. As Ruth Kirschstein, M.D., acting associate director for research on women's health at the NIH, observed, "Then maybe women would be in better shape and the quality of their lives might be improved."

OVERCOMING DISCRIMINATION

Finally, attitudes toward women and their health have begun to change. The first evidence of bias in the diagnosis and treatment of heart disease was published in 1987. Although critics found flaws in that study, it raised eyebrows, fired debate, and inspired additional investigations. By 1991, the indicting evidence was incontrovertible. In addition, women, who held 31 of 535 congressional seats as of 1990, are gradually acquiring a stronger voice and greater support in government. Women are also beginning to assume powerful positions in medical research. With Antonia Novello as Surgeon General of the United States and Bernadine Healy as the director of the National Institutes of Health, the government's two highest medical positions are held by women for the first time in history. Bernadine Healy, formerly chief of research at the Cleveland Clinic and a past president of the American Heart Association, is particularly invested in effecting change.

In June 1990, the GAO issued its report to Congress, and the following month the Congressional Caucus for Women introduced the Women's Health Equity Act to remedy the problem. Among other provisions, the act provided for the Office of Research on Women's Health at NIH to coordinate the interdisciplinary efforts among the various institutes and thereby to close the research gap as expediently as possible. The effort was supported by unusually vigorous media coverage, which raised awareness among the general public and health professionals.

Although Congress adjourned that summer before the Women's Health Equity Act could be enacted into law, NIH voluntarily established the Office of Research in Women's Health in September 1990 to make sure that women are appropriately represented in studies and to coordinate interdisciplinary research activities. In contrast to the halfhearted spirit with which NIH implemented the Public Health Policy Task Force recommendations in 1986, the new office swiftly sponsored training sessions for all staff involved with funding grants. NIH strengthened its resolve to fund only those proposals that include women and minorities proportionately or that provide compelling justification for exemption. NIH has revised grant application forms to assure getting the information they seek. And they have begun studies on cholesterol-lowering drugs in older people—men and women—as well as some pilot studies in other areas.

In addition, in April 1991, Dr. Healy announced the Healthy Women's Study, the first large-scale study of American women's health. Designed to determine the causes of cancer, heart disease, and osteoporosis in women, this ten-year initiative will be "the most definitive, far-reaching study of women's health ever undertaken," according to Dr. Healy, and will analyze how the diseases are affected by hormone replacement, quitting smoking, diet, and exercise. The research will be coordinated by the Office of Research on Women's Health and will involve six of the National Institutes of Health. NIH also held two fact-finding conferences later in 1991 and a large conference early in 1992 to identify specific needs in heart disease research and establish an interdisciplinary approach to meeting them. Dr. Nanette Wenger, chair of the 1992 conference, estimates that it will take five to ten years to ask the right questions, develop the studies, and launch them.

Separate from NIH, the *Journal of the American Medical Association* devoted an entire issue to women's health in the summer of 1992. The American Medical Association, together with the American Dental Association, have also pledged a Women's Health Campaign, an effort designed to feature a range of educational and motivational activities. By all indications, it is suddenly socially and politically prudent to address the problems of women's health.

Perhaps the best indication of the changing times is reflected in research on aspirin. In disclosing the health bias against women, exposé after exposé alluded to a study of 22,000 men and zero women documenting that an aspirin taken every other day helps prevent heart disease. The allusions were so frequent that the Physicians Health Study became synonymous with discrimination. Ironically, Charles Hennekens, M.D., the Harvard researcher who led this study and one of the principal investigators of the Nurses Health Study, had been trying for five years to get funding to repeat the work in 45,000 female nurses. Available data had already documented that women who survived a heart attack or stroke or who had severe angina could be helped by aspirin. Dr. Hennekens wanted clear proof that the drug could also help women before a heart attack. Since evidence suggests that races and ethnic groups react uniquely to drugs, he proposed looking separately at how well aspirin works in whites, blacks, Hispanics, and other minorities.

Some animal studies suggest that women's bodies might react very differently to aspirin than men's. Because of hormonal differences, a dose of aspirin that benefits men may harm women. Yet NIH rejected Dr. Hennekens's grant proposal three times. Each time he was told there was insufficient justification to study women separately.

In February 1991, Dr. Hennekens finally won preliminary approval for his work. The following month, NIH became aware of two new studies, the results of which were promising but inconclusive. In contrast to these, which implied that aspirin might help women, a third study of older women found just the opposite. According to Dr. Hennekens, the available research provided information about women comparable to what was known about men in 1981, before the Physicians Health Study began. The only way to get the definitive word on benefit and risk as well as precise guidance on dosage was with a clinical experiment comparable to the one conducted on men. Nevertheless, in light of the new research, NIH requested that Dr. Hennekens defend his intentions more vigorously. He did, and in July, the National Heart, Lung, and Blood Institute advisory committee rejected his $10 million proposal again. Although the committee acknowledged that such a study deserved "the highest priority," they found technical problems with Dr. Hennekens's proposal.

Then Dr. Claude J. Lenfant, director of the Heart, Lung, and Blood Institute, overruled the advisory group. Dr. Hennekens got his money.

If there is any obstacle to closing the research gap, it is money. The studies on heart disease in men cost at least $20 million. Replicating them in women, with the necessary increases in study sizes, will be very expensive. The ten-year Women's Health Initiative, announced in April 1991, is estimated to cost $500 million.

While the national financial crisis makes money a valid concern, those committed to promoting research on women's health are optimistic. In fiscal 1992, Congress raised its budget for women's health research by $240 million. Included is a fivefold increase for breast cancer research ($133 million compared to $48 million ten years ago) and a better than threefold increase in allocation for ovarian cancer ($20 million compared to $6.5 million in 1987–88).

In August 1991, NIH began its first major investigation of aging in women. In April 1992, NIH announced a 16,000-participant study of tamoxifen, a drug that has been treating breast cancer successfully for a decade. The goal of the new research is to assess this drug's ability to prevent breast cancer, heart disease, and osteoporosis. All told, the 1992 allocations will permit research involving 80,000 women to begin by 1993 and continue through the decade.

Public policy experts feel confident that women's research will continue to get the funding it needs. Legislators, lobbyists, and researchers agree that public awareness and outrage were critical first steps and now money will follow. Finally, the political climate is ripe.

TAKE ACTION

Under the best of circumstances, it will take years to close the research gap and spread the truth about heart disease in women. In the meantime, you can protect yourself by assuming an active partnership with a knowledgeable physician who is committed to giving women good care.

- To fulfill your part in this partnership, understand the unique dynamics of heart disease in women—Chapter 2.
- Identify your personal risks—Chapter 3.

- If you are at risk or develop symptoms, get a reliable and comprehensive diagnosis—Chapter 4.
- If necessary, get definitive treatment and emotional support—Chapters 5, 6, 7, and 8.
- Begin to reduce your personal risk. Evaluate the merits of hormone replacement therapy, adopt a low-fat diet, exercise regularly, don't smoke, and keep your stress in check—Chapters 9 and 10.
- Start today to live heart-smart so that you can have a longer, fuller life.

CHAPTER 2

What Is Heart Disease and What Are Its Symptoms?

The call came in to the Arizona Heart Institute at 12:35 A.M. "We have a match—a heart to fit a one-hundred-and-ten-pound woman, blood type A." This heart, still beating, was stopped, carefully removed from the accident victim's brain-dead body, and placed on ice in a picnic cooler. Three hours later, having been rushed halfway across the country, the cold, still heart was lifted from its bed of ice and set into the open, readied chest of forty-three-year-old Margaret Roth, whose own heart, diseased beyond hope, had been removed. As Margaret's body warmed her new heart, it came back to life. Within seconds its beat was regular and robust. One person's tragedy had become another's salvation.

On another day in another place, another middle-aged woman began her daily aerobics regime. Fifteen minutes into a routine she had performed several times a week for over five years, without warning she turned pale and collapsed. Despite her youth—she was only forty—vigor, and apparent good health, she succumbed to a heart attack so massive that it killed her instantly.

What supreme irony: The heart is so frail that a tiny clot of blood can stifle it in an instant, yet durable enough to survive a plane ride in a picnic cooler. It is subject to a wide range of diseases and maladies—some of trivial consequence or merely annoying, others life threatening. This chapter explains how the heart works and what can happen when it stops functioning properly.

Tenacious and enduring, the heart empties and fills, empties and fills, one hundred thousand times every day, more than two and a half billion times over the span of a normal life. In the process, it dispatches more than two thousand gallons of oxygen- and nutrient-bearing blood to all the cells of the body. Propelled by a self-energized electrical system, the strong muscular walls of this four-chambered pump contract, the valves between them open, and the blood progresses on its circuit. If a drop of blood could be tagged as it exchanges carbon dioxide for oxygen in the lung, it would be possible to watch it begin its journey.

THE INTRICACIES OF CIRCULATION

Newly replenished blood leaves the lungs and fills the small, triangular chamber in the upper-left quadrant of the heart (Figure 2-1). This is the *left atrium*, which holds the blood until an electrical impulse squeezes the muscle, unlocking the *mitral valve* at the base of the chamber. As the floodgates open, blood rushes into the *left ventricle* below, the largest, strongest, and most important compartment of the pump. When this ventricle constricts in response to electrical charge, the blood surges through the *aortic valve* into the avenues of the circulatory system. From the *aorta*, or main artery, it travels a complex route to near and distant points, where it exchanges oxygen and other nutrients for carbon dioxide and other wastes. By the time the blood wends its way through the smaller arteries and minuscule capillaries, by the time it continues through the complex system of veins and returns to the heart, the blood will have traveled 12,400 miles. On its return, it enters the heart's right side: first the *right atrium*, then the *right ventricle* below, and finally back to the lungs, where it gets rid of accumulated carbon dioxide and picks up a fresh supply of oxygen so that the process can begin again (Figure 2-2).

DISORDERS OF THE PUMP

With such a complex pumping mechanism, any number of problems can occur to compromise its efficiency. The heart can grow weak and lose pumping power, a condition known as *congestive heart failure*. The

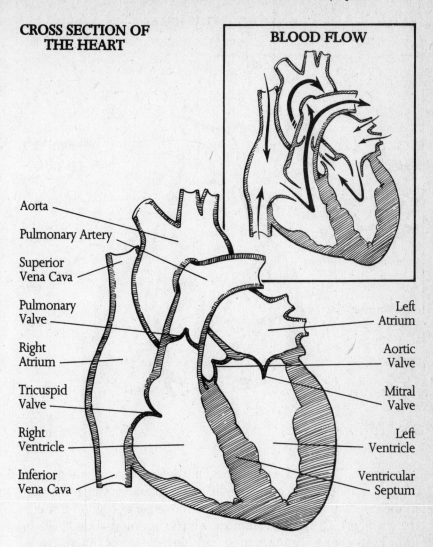

CROSS SECTION OF THE HEART

BLOOD FLOW

Aorta

Pulmonary Artery

Superior Vena Cava

Pulmonary Valve

Right Atrium

Tricuspid Valve

Right Ventricle

Inferior Vena Cava

Left Atrium

Aortic Valve

Mitral Valve

Left Ventricle

Ventricular Septum

FIGURE 2-1.

electrical system can malfunction, causing palpitations, or *arrhythmias.* The heart can beat too slowly (*bradycardia*), too quickly (*tachycardia*), or erratically. A hole in the wall between the chambers, usually congenital and usually between the two atria (*atrial septal defect*) can compromise the integrity of each of these chambers, permitting blood to slosh between them, mixing oxygen-rich blood with its waste-laden

ANATOMY OF THE HEART

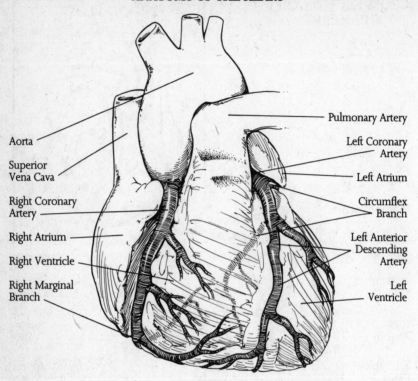

Aorta

Superior
Vena Cava

Right Coronary
Artery

Right Atrium

Right Ventricle

Right Marginal
Branch

Pulmonary Artery

Left Coronary
Artery

Left Atrium

Circumflex
Branch

Left Anterior
Descending
Artery

Left
Ventricle

FIGURE 2-2.

counterpart. The valves, too, can become defective. As a consequence of aging or illness, they can grow stiff and calcified, causing narrowing of the opening (*stenosis*), inhibiting the movement of blood through the chambers. Occasionally tumors, which are almost always benign, form in the heart chamber; these can plug the valves. Alternatively, valves damaged by disease or congenital defect can leak (*insufficiency*), compromising the vertical separation of the chambers and diminishing the efficiency of blood flow. Into this category falls the common, often debilitating, but rarely serious condition called *mitral valve prolapse*, which afflicts more women than men. Far more serious—because of both its high incidence and potential danger—is damage to the heart muscle, the consequence of a heart attack, or *myocardial infarction*. Heart attacks occur when the *coronary arteries*, located on its outer surface, become blocked.

Coronary Circulation

Although the chambers of the heart fill with blood repeatedly, the muscle gets little nourishment from within the chambers. Rather, the organ is fed by the first network of arteries that fork off the aorta just above the aortic valve. Positioned this way, the coronary arteries have first dibs on outbound oxygen-rich blood. As each subsequent bolus of blood bursts through the aortic valve, some of the blood already in the aorta and destined for distant parts is forced immediately into the coronary arteries. Thus, cardiologists like to say, "First the heart feeds itself."

When the coronary arteries are healthy, blood flows through them easily. During physical or emotional stress, when the heart pumps more quickly and demands additional nourishment, healthy, unobstructed coronary arteries dilate to meet this need. Several conditions can impede coronary circulation. Occasionally the problem occurs because the tiniest capillaries that branch off the coronary arteries fail to dilate. The condition, called *syndrome X* because little is known about it, does not cause heart attacks and so is not life threatening. Somewhat more frequently, one or more of the coronary arteries spontaneously constrict in spasm, a condition called *Prinzmetal's* or *variant angina*. Spasms seldom last long enough to cause a heart attack.

By far the most common cause of trouble occurs when the coronary arteries become encrusted with debris, which stiffens the artery wall and narrows the channel within. Like disabled automobiles that block a roadway and cause the backup of traffic, debris in the artery impedes blood flow. The bottleneck, which prevents the heart muscle from receiving adequate nourishment during periods of physical and/or emotional stress, causes oxygen insufficiency, or *ischemia*, and is characterized by chest pain called *angina* (Figure 2-3). Should a blood clot or loose piece of plaque (see below) lodge in this narrowing, blood flow is entirely blocked. Unless it is quickly restored, the portion of heart muscle fed by the affected artery dies from lack of oxygen and is replaced by scar tissue. This is a heart attack.

HARDENING OF THE ARTERIES

How do the coronary arteries become blocked?

The encrusting of the arteries—not just the coronary arteries but other major arteries in the torso, limbs, and neck as well—is a gradual

ISCHEMIA AND MYOCARDIAL INFARCTION

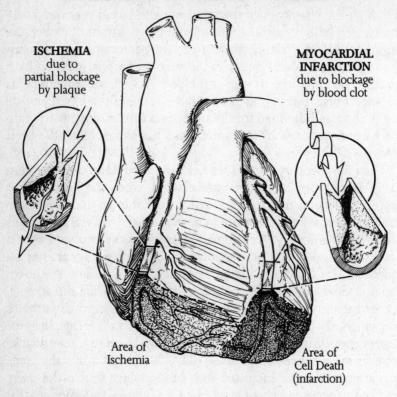

ISCHEMIA
due to
partial blockage
by plaque

**MYOCARDIAL
INFARCTION**
due to blockage
by blood clot

Area of
Ischemia

Area of
Cell Death
(infarction)

FIGURE 2-3.

process called *atherosclerosis* (Figure 2-4). The primary villain is cholesterol, a soft, waxy, fatlike substance that collects on the lining of the artery walls. Our bodies need some cholesterol to manufacture essential substances such as sex hormones, muscle membranes, and collagen, which helps keep our skin from sagging and supports other body tissues. In excess, however, cholesterol remains in the blood, setting the stage for atherosclerosis.

This process has been studied in millions of autopsies of patients young and old from fourteen countries and nineteen racial groups. This enormous body of research documents that fatty streaks on the artery wall, the first signs of atherosclerosis, can begin to appear by age three. In cultures where coronary-prone behaviors don't exist,

ATHEROSCLEROSIS—HARDENING OF THE ARTERIES

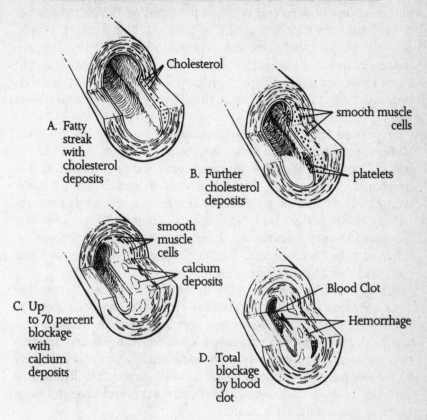

A. Fatty streak with cholesterol deposits

Cholesterol

B. Further cholesterol deposits

smooth muscle cells

platelets

C. Up to 70 percent blockage with calcium deposits

smooth muscle cells

calcium deposits

D. Total blockage by blood clot

Blood Clot

Hemorrhage

FIGURE 2-4.

these fatty streaks cause no harm. But in industrialized nations, where life-style is characterized by such perils as rich diet, emotional stress, and sedentary habits, the fat circulating in the blood is drawn to these streaks, where it begins to wreak havoc.

As the fatty streaks etch a foothold, they injure the artery wall, tearing up its surface and disrupting the blood flow. Like rocks in a riverbed, which can churn up the flowing water and trap debris floating downstream, turbulence in the bloodstream disturbs the flow and attracts the fats circulating in the blood. The fats adhere to the established streaks and the atherosclerotic process advances.

Gradually, mounds develop. They bulge into the arterial canal and, little by little, they dam it up. As time goes on the *plaque*, soft and fibrous at first, stiffens and weakens the artery wall. The arteries become brittle and more vulnerable to tears and hemorrhages. Worse, once the plaque calcifies, pieces can break off and get lodged downstream. Plaque also invites the blood to clot upon it. These clots can come loose and travel downstream as well. Thus, once plaque develops, especially if it obstructs more than 70 percent of the vessel, heart attacks can occur.

In women and in men, the coronary arteries clog up in similar fashion. Yet the two genders are surprisingly different, and we're not just talking about the reproductive organs. Largely because of sex hormones, which assert themselves early in gestation, men's and women's bodies develop differently and behave differently throughout life. (This is discussed more fully in Chapter 3.) Because their biochemical environments are different, men and women exhibit different patterns of disease, they perform differently on diagnostic tests, and they respond differently to treatment.

Where heart disease is concerned, it is not unusual for men to collapse from a heart attack without any prior hint that their coronary arteries are blocked. However, this scenario is rare in women, who are much more likely to experience a period of angina first. In addition, women are more likely to develop heart failure and less likely to recover fully from a heart attack or heart surgery. Finally, for reasons not entirely understood, chest pain is more elusive and enigmatic in women than it is in men.

RECOGNIZING HEART PAIN

When the coronary circulation cannot meet the heart's need for oxygen-rich blood, chest pain or shortness of breath occurs as the body's way of crying, "Stop." Classically—though not always and, unfortunately, less reliably in women than in men—angina appears as a dull pain deep beneath the breastbone or as a band across the chest. The pain often radiates to the left arm and/or shoulder, neck, jaw, teeth. It can also travel down the back, and it can be accompanied by nausea, sweating, and shortness of breath. People with heart disease commonly say it's more a tightness, heaviness, or squeezing sensation than outright pain, and it is frequently misinterpreted as indigestion.

In its early stages, angina usually comes with physical or emotional stress and may last only moments. It usually stops when you stop exerting yourself, signaling that your circulation is adequate when you're inactive and relaxed. Surveys reveal that this pattern is less consistent in women than in men, but no one knows why. Perhaps, since women and their doctors do not commonly think in terms of women having heart disease, they overlook or misidentify these early symptoms. When this happens, the condition progresses undetected.

As blockages grow larger, angina characteristically becomes more severe and erratic, a variation called *unstable angina.* At this point, angina may come without provocation, perhaps when you're lying in bed at night or sitting and reading during the day. It may come variably with exertion or during rest. Many women describe the pain they feel in ways consistent with unstable angina, suggesting that, for whatever reason, they first become aware of their chest discomfort or have it diagnosed only after it reaches this more advanced state.

Ultimately, a heart attack may occur. Classically, heart attacks strike with crushing chest pain, which radiates to the arm, neck, jaw, teeth, and/or back. Unlike angina, it does not respond to rest or the medications that treat angina. During a heart attack, patients often have trouble breathing. They commonly experience palpitations, feel nauseated and/or vomit, break out in a cold sweat, turn pale, and feel weak and apprehensive.

SILENT HEART DISEASE

However, some people, especially women, develop heart disease and even suffer heart attacks without realizing it, a phenomenon called *silent heart disease.* In the Framingham population, 35 percent of heart attacks in women, compared to 28 percent in men, went unrecognized. Half of these were completely pain free, according to William Kannel, M.D., former director of the study; the other half appeared disguised as indigestion, ulcers, arthritis, or other conditions.

Cardiac testing has demonstrated that ischemia and life-threatening irregular heart rhythms can occur without symptoms of any kind. Plaque can develop insidiously and impede blood flow substantially enough to inflict tiny injury after tiny injury upon the heart muscle. Ultimately a massive heart attack can strike and snuff out life without so much as a twinge.

Sometimes, patients experience symptoms and their physicians misdiagnose them. Patients sometimes suspect they have heart trouble only to be told by their doctors that they are suffering from anxiety, indigestion, or another condition that produces similar symptoms.

Still other times patients themselves misinterpret their symptoms. This error may result from our natural human tendency to diagnose ourselves. Once we decide what's probably wrong, we subconsciously filter out any sensations that don't conform to our diagnosis. If patients don't expect to have heart disease, they may not recognize it when it strikes.

Perhaps it was this psychological mechanism that kept Rose Mercer from going to the doctor. When Rose's discomfort began one evening, she thought she was having indigestion and tried to quell it, but the antacids didn't work; her pain subsided slightly, but it never quite went away. In bed that night, she needed two pillows to compensate for her shortness of breath. Still, she didn't seek medical attention for two days, by which time she'd already sustained permanent damage from a heart attack.

While Rose may have been convinced that she was suffering from indigestion, it is also possible that she feared otherwise and was experiencing another natural human tendency: to deny the obvious. Denial, the inclination to consciously or unconsciously ignore what we are feeling out of fear, is a well-recognized defense mechanism that protects people from threatening information. Research documents that deniers have less heart pain than those who cope in other ways.

Experts agree that, regardless of its cause, silent heart disease is an important component of women's discouraging heart-disease profile. When women have a heart attack, they are nearly 50 percent more likely than men to die before they leave the hospital, in part because they delay getting immediate treatment. If they do recover enough to go home, they are more likely than men to suffer a second attack or die during the next two years. In addition, when ischemia goes untreated—that is, when part of the heart muscle is chronically deprived of oxygen—heart failure often follows, and heart failure makes subsequent heart attacks more dangerous and increases risk from invasive treatments such as bypass surgery.

WOMEN'S CONFUSING SYMPTOMS

To complicate the matter, women sometimes have symptoms of heart disease that don't fit the formula. Some experience not shortness of breath but a sensation akin to inhaling cold air. Others complain only of weakness and lethargy. One woman's chest pain asserted itself as a hot poker stabbing her between her breasts, diagonally up across her chest, and deep into her left armpit. Another found her chest pain traveling down her right arm, not the left, as it classically does. A third first experienced angina as back pain, but later felt it as a deep aching and throbbing in her right biceps (Figure 2-5).

Moreover, for reasons not fully understood, women frequently experience inconsequential chest pains and fleeting rhythm disturbances periodically from the time they are very young. All of a sudden, the heart seems to jump into the throat, skip, or take off in a gallop. But the episode is over in seconds. Young women also commonly experience momentary sharp twinges in the center of their chests when they move or breathe. Sometimes they complain of burning or aching in the front of the chest, usually in the area of the pectoral muscles, which are located midway between the breast and the collarbone. These sensations usually reflect muscular problems that can come from carrying a heavy shoulder bag or holding children, either on the hip or in a baby carrier. Heavy-breasted women in particular seem burdened by such pain. Sometimes women wind up with a charley horse in the front of the chest that lasts for days after they exercise too strenuously or throw themselves into a workout without warming up. And occasionally, women encounter *Tietze's syndrome*, an inflammation of the cartilage between the breastbone and the ribs, which can cause pain on the left side around the second and third ribs. This pain is hard to suppress and sometimes lasts for weeks and weeks, only to return several times.

Anxiety, too, can produce harmless chest pain. Usually it waxes and wanes, rarely feels unrelenting or intense, and is clearly associated with stressful experiences or emotions. Women say it comes and goes for hours at a time. The pain may be accompanied by hyperventilation, which in turn can cause a tingling or slight numbness in the fingertips, on the tongue, around the mouth, and sometimes down the legs.

To further confuse the issue, hiatal hernias, gallbladder disease, and other less serious conditions often look alarmingly like heart pain.

FIGURE 2-5.

HEART ATTACKS DON'T ALWAYS FEEL THE SAME

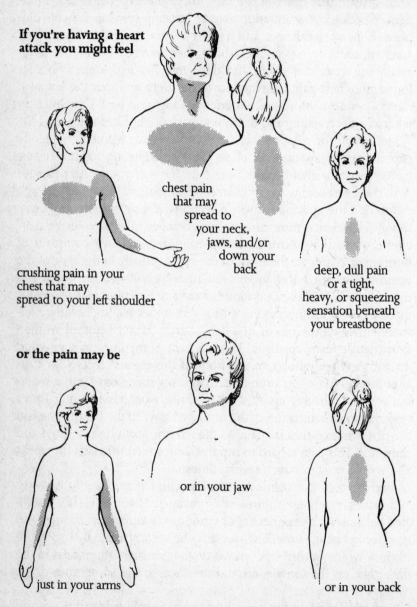

If you're having a heart attack you might feel

chest pain that may spread to your neck, jaws, and/or down your back

crushing pain in your chest that may spread to your left shoulder

deep, dull pain or a tight, heavy, or squeezing sensation beneath your breastbone

or the pain may be

just in your arms

or in your jaw

or in your back

One patient, age seventy-seven and recovering from a year full of medical catastrophes, was sure she was having a heart attack when she felt classic chest pain, which radiated into her jaw, neck, back, and left arm. Diagnosis: spasm of the esophagus. Another patient had identical symptoms and was rushed to the hospital for emergency treatment of a heart attack. But tests revealed she was having a gall-bladder attack. A third patient complained of an intense, dull heaviness between the breasts almost constantly. Her diagnosis: hiatal hernia.

IS YOUR HEART PAIN REAL?

If heart pain is so hard to identify, how can you tell if you're having it?

Good question.

"Heart disease is a tough nut to crack," admits Raymond Bahr, M.D., director of critical care at St. Agnes Hospital in Baltimore, Maryland. In 1981, he created a special chest pain emergency room at St. Agnes, where a better-safe-than-sorry attitude guarantees immediate attention even for patients with ambiguous symptoms.

Patients commonly confess that they equivocate because they have trouble evaluating their pain. They also report they are sometimes ridiculed when they go to the emergency room only to find nothing is seriously wrong.

One patient complained, "My physician told me there are good chest pains and bad chest pains. How am I supposed to be able to tell?"

Dr. Marc Silver, acting chief of cardiology at Chicago's Michael Reese Hospital, responds that putting this kind of burden on the patient is unconscionable. "No one should make you feel like a jerk if you go to the emergency room unnecessarily. If they can't give you clear clues, then it's their job to take care of you." The consequences of negligence can be profound.

If, on the other hand, emergency treatment with clot-busting drugs such as streptokinase or tissue plasminogen activator (tPA) is instituted within four to six hours after symptoms begin, the attack can often be halted in progress, before it damages the muscle (see Chapter 6). When caught this way, a heart attack becomes merely a revelation, and not a disaster.

The best news for women is that heart attacks rarely strike without warning, as they do in men. So if women have a strategy for dealing with symptoms, they can begin medical care before they run into trouble.

TAKE ACTION

Heart attack symptoms are often equivocal, but having a clear strategy can mean the difference between life and death.

Know the early signals of heart attack:
- uncomfortable pressure, fullness, squeezing, or pain in the chest, usually lasting longer than two minutes
- pain radiating to the shoulders, neck, jaw, arms, or back
- dizziness, fainting, sweating, nausea, shortness of breath, or weakness

None of these symptoms certifies that a heart attack is in progress, but the more symptoms you have, the more likely it is.

If you know you have heart disease, *presume you are having a heart attack if:*
- You think you have indigestion, but your pain does not respond to antacids.
- You develop angina that does not respond to nitroglycerin.

If you suspect you are having a heart attack:
- Stop whatever you're doing and sit down or lie down.
- Take up to three nitroglycerin tablets—one at a time at five-minute intervals or as prescribed by your doctor. If the pain does not go away, call 911 or your local emergency number immediately.
- If you do not have nitroglycerin and have had symptoms for two minutes or more, call 911 or your local emergency number immediately.
- If you can get to the hospital faster by car, have someone drive you. Do not drive yourself to the hospital!
- When you get to the hospital, do not permit emergency room personnel to keep you waiting.

- DO NOT MINIMIZE YOUR SYMPTOMS. DO NOT DELAY. Waiting more than fifteen minutes to see if the pain goes away can result in permanent damage to your heart. At worst, it can cost you your life.

If you are with someone who appears to be having a heart attack:
- Do not permit the person to persuade you that her problem is inconsequential.
- Call 911 or your local emergency number immediately. If you can get the patient to the hospital more quickly by driving, do so without delay.
- While waiting for assistance, make the person comfortable, usually by making her lie down with her head slightly elevated.
- Check for medical alert tags around the person's wrist or neck and follow any pertinent emergency instructions. Call these tags to the attention of medical personnel when they arrive.
- If you have been properly trained and the need arises, begin CPR and keep it going until help arrives.

If you have never been diagnosed with heart disease but develop any of the following symptoms, consider the possibility that you have angina, make an appointment with your doctor, and arrange for a cardiac screening:
- chest pain that comes with physical exertion and eases with rest
- chest pain that is brought on by emotional stress
- new or unusual shortness of breath—if you suddenly find you're winded after climbing a flight of stairs when you used to be able to take the same flight of stairs in stride, for example
- indigestion, particularly if indigestion is unusual for you, if it does not respond to antacids, or if you do not associate its occurrence with eating

To guard against silent heart disease, all women need regular medical checkups from an understanding physician who practices good preventive medicine and accepts the truth that women can get heart disease. Regardless of your age, if your score on the heart test in the next chapter is 33 or above, you should recognize your high-risk status and have annual checkups, including an exercise stress test, even if you have no symptoms. If you are healthy, take birth control pills, or are over the age of forty-five, you should also have yearly checkups. If you are younger than forty-five, do not use oral contraceptives, and score 15 or below on the heart test, medical exams every five years are sufficient. Youngsters even in their teens need to have their blood pressure and, perhaps, their cholesterol screened. (Cholesterol screening in children and teenagers is controversial. See Chapter 10.)

Heart disease need not remain the number-one threat to women's health. With diligent preventive tactics, persistent pursuit of diagnosis, and prompt, aggressive treatment, we can beat the killer.

CHAPTER 3

Are You at Risk for Heart Disease?

How susceptible to heart disease are you? Knowing can save your life.

Early in its history, the Framingham study showed how certain conditions, known as *risk factors*, increased people's vulnerability to heart disease. The concept, which pertains to probability based on the statistical analysis of huge populations, does not imply clear-cut cause and effect. In other words, if your blood pressure and cholesterol are high, there is no guarantee that you will get heart disease. Nor is there any guarantee that you will avoid trouble if you lower your risk. But if your risk is low, you are less likely to develop disease than someone whose risk is high.

A QUICK TEST TO ASSESS YOUR RISK

To help you assess your personal vulnerability, researchers at the Arizona Heart Institute have compiled the following survey based on the unique dynamics of risk in women. The test covers those risk factors that have been proven time and again to influence women's risk in a predictable way. You will notice that it does not include some of the risk factors we discuss later in the chapter, notably tri-glycerides, fibrinogen, and socioeconomic status. At best, this kind of written test is a rough measure; the statisticians who devised this survey attempted to strengthen its validity by including only those factors whose degree of influence has been repeatedly, and therefore reliably, confirmed.

Take the test and add up your score.

ARIZONA HEART INSTITUTE'S HEART TEST FOR WOMEN

Age   **Score**

    51 and over 5

    35 to 50..................................... 2   *5*

    34 and under 0

Family History

    If you have parents, brothers, or sisters who
    have had a heart attack, stroke, or heart bypass
    surgery at:

    Age 55 or before 5

    Age 56 or after 3   *3*

    None or don't know 0

Personal History

    Have you had:

    a heart attack 20

    angina, heart bypass surgery, angioplasty,

    stroke, or blood vessel surgery 10   *10*

    none of the above 0

Smoking

    Current smoker: how many cigarettes per day?

    5 or more.................................. 20

    4 or fewer 10

    If you are a smoker currently taking oral
    contraceptives and are under 35 years old,
    add 2; if 35 years old or over, add 5.

Previous smoker who quit less than two years
ago: How many cigarettes did you smoke?

5 or more 10
4 or fewer 5
Never smoked or quit more than two years ago 0

0

Blood Pressure

If you have had your blood pressure taken in the
last year, was it:

Elevated or high (either or both readings above
160/95) 6
Borderline (between 140/90 and 160/95) 3
Normal (below 140/90) or don't know 0

3

Blood Fats

If you have had your cholesterol and blood fat
levels checked in the last year, score your risk
here:

over 240 mg/dL 6
200 to 240 mg/dL 3
cholesterol under 200 mg/dL 0
Are your HDL's lower than 45? . . . . Add 1
0

OR

If you know your cholesterol-to-HDL ratio, use
this section to score your risk:

7.1 and above 6
3.6–7.0 3
3.5 or below 0 *0*

OR

If you do not know your blood fat levels, use this
section to score your risk:

Which of the following best describes your eating
pattern:

high fat: red meat and/or fried foods daily, more
than seven eggs per week, and regular consumption of butter, whole milk, and cheese 6
medium fat: red meat and/or fried foods four to
six times per week, four to seven eggs weekly,
regular use of margarine, vegetable oils, and/or
low-fat dairy products 3

low fat: poultry, fish, and little or no red meat, fried foods, or saturated fats, fewer than three eggs per week, minimal margarine and vegetable oils, primarily non-fat dairy products, skim milk, and skim milk products 0

USE SCORE FROM ONLY ONE SECTION

0

Diabetes

If you have diabetes (blood sugar above 140 mg/DL), your age when you found out:

40 or before................................. 6
41 or older.................................. 4
Do not have diabetes........................ 0

0

Body Mass

Calculate your body mass index with the following formula:

weight (pounds): _145_ × 0.45 = _65.30_ (W)
height (inches): _54_ × 0.025 = _1.35_ (H)

Now divide your weight W by the square of your height (H × H) or W/H × H = body mass index (BMI)

Example: a woman is 120 pounds and 5 feet 6 inches tall:

$120 \times 0.45 = 54 = W$ $66 \times 0.025 = 1.65 = H$
$W/H \times H = 54/1.65 \times 1.65 = 54/2.72 = 19.8$ BMI

If your BMI is 27 or greater 2
If your BMI is below 27...................... 0

0

Now measure your waist and hips and divide your waist measurement by your hip girth. For example, your waist is 26 and your hips are 36: 26/36 = 0.7.

If your waist-to-hip ratio is 0.8 or greater....... 1
If your ratio is 0.79 or lower.................. 0

0

Menopause

If you have undergone natural menopause, your age at its start:

41 or older................................... 1
40 or younger 2

If you have had a total hysterectomy, your age
when it was done

41 or older	1
40 or younger	3

If you take an oral estrogen
supplement . . . . subtract 2
If you are still menstruating . . . . subtract 1

Exercise

Do you engage in any aerobic activity, such as
brisk walking, jogging, bicycling, or swimming for
more than 20 minutes:

Less than once a week	6
One or two times a week	3
Three or more times a week	0

0

Stress

Are you easily angered and frustrated

Most of the time	6
Some of the time	3
Rarely	0

3

TOTAL SCORE

Interpreting Your Score

If your total score is 33 or above, you are in danger of heart disease.
You must start lowering your risk immediately (see Chapter 10). Make
an appointment with your physician right away. Be sure he or she
knows about your risk profile and schedules an appropriate cardiac
screening. No matter what your age, if you develop chest pain, do
not ignore it.

If your score is between 16 and 32, realize that you are vulnerable.
Step up your efforts to lower your risk further with healthy diet and
exercise (see Chapter 10). If you are over age fifty and develop chest
pain, be aware that you may be having angina. Whether or not you
have symptoms, an annual checkup is a good idea.

If your score is 15 or below, your risk is probably low. Live in heart-
smart style and continue to have blood pressure and cholesterol
checks periodically to make sure that your risk stays low.

What do these risk factors mean? Some are just fortune's roll of the dice—you can't change your parents, for example, so you can't change the role of heredity in your risk of heart disease. But you can stay in charge of many of these risk factors. Let's discuss them in turn.

HIGH BLOOD PRESSURE

If you have high blood pressure, or *hypertension*, you have something in common with fifty-eight million other Americans, half of them women, and most of these black. While men younger than fifty-five are more susceptible to the condition than are women of the same age, the balance flips by age sixty-five. From then on, two out of every three women are afflicted.

Harriet Silber, a bouncy octogenarian, is a typical person with hypertension. At four feet ten inches, she has always had trouble keeping her weight in line. As often happens when women are overweight, she developed high blood pressure in her forties. The condition caused no symptoms for years. A longtime widow, she raised her children alone and led an active social life. But hypertension ultimately took its toll. When Harriet was eighty, she developed angina and by eighty-two needed bypass surgery.

High blood pressure tends to run in families. It is exacerbated by obesity, and it is associated with diabetes and regular alcohol use. A few patients develop high blood pressure as the by-product of kidney disease, thyroid dysfunction, or an abnormal genetic condition. In young women, high blood pressure is sometimes caused by oral contraceptives or pregnancy. But for the most part, it has no known cause and appears without symptoms.

Yet it is clearly dangerous. Elevated blood pressure causes the blood to pound against the artery walls with each beat of the heart. The reverberating force increases the heart's workload, causing the muscle to enlarge and weaken over time, and thus setting the stage for heart failure. This force also injures the artery walls, stimulating the blood's repair mechanism and inclination to clot. Even if your blood pressure is just a little high, you are doubly vulnerable to stroke and significantly more susceptible to heart attack and kidney disease than you would be with normal blood pressure. Hence, this condition has earned the label "silent killer."

The latest data on high blood pressure in women comes out of the Mayo Clinic. After your other risk factors are statistically eliminated, if you are between ages forty and fifty-nine and have high blood pressure, you are likely to encounter angina, heart attack, or sudden death at five times the normal rate. If your blood pressure is brought into the normal range by diet, exercise, and/or medication, most of this risk disappears.

The numbers in the blood pressure reading reflect the greatest force the blood exerts against the arteries while the heart is contracting and the lowest pressure that occurs while it is relaxing. These numbers are expressed as a fraction, the former or *systolic* pressure written as the numerator and the latter or *diastolic* pressure as the denominator. Normal blood pressure is classified as 120/80, borderline hypertension as up to 160/95, and high blood pressure as anything above. A variant type of high blood pressure, called *isolated systolic hypertension*, occurs when the pressure caused by the contracting heart consistently registers 160 or more while the minimum pressure during the heart's relaxation phase remains lower than 95. Systolic hypertension afflicts more women than men and constitutes the most common variety of high blood pressure among the elderly.

We first learned about the merits of controlling blood pressure through the Hypertension Detection and Follow-Up Program. Launched in 1973 with 11,000 women and men, this landmark study measured the effectiveness of a specific sequence of treatments. In this study, treatment helped black women most, saving 28 percent of their lives, compared to 18 percent of black men and 15 percent of white men. Curiously, the study showed no benefit for white women or participants in the twenty to forty-nine age group, a finding that probably tells more about the nature of statistics than the treatment of high blood pressure. Since high blood pressure kills few people in these categories, these two subgroups would have to be represented in enormous numbers for the research to produce statistically significant results. Consequently, experts suspect that the study's design obscured the true impact of treatment on white women and all men and women aged twenty to forty-nine. Nevertheless, it did demonstrate that effective treatment of high blood pressure has profound benefits. (For more on the treatment of high blood pressure, see Chapter 10.)

High blood pressure is especially widespread among African-Americans. Some studies suggest a genetic link between pigmentation and susceptibility, but racism, together with limited social and economic opportunities, probably deserves more blame. Poor eating habits and obesity develop, and diabetes and hypertension follow. Chronic frustration has also been implicated. These observations take on particular meaning in light of 1990 statistics confirming that poor blacks in America are dying prematurely from a distressing range of treatable illnesses, hypertensive heart disease among them (see the section on socioeconomic status as a risk factor later in this chapter.)

CHOLESTEROL AND TRIGLYCERIDES

The primary culprit of atherosclerosis, excess cholesterol circulating in the bloodstream, develops in two ways. First, we consume it when we eat animal products: meat, fish, eggs, and dairy. The cholesterol contained in these foods is absorbed directly into the blood from the small intestine. Second, it is manufactured in the liver from other dietary fats we consume, primarily saturated fats, which come from both animal and vegetable foodstuffs. Although margarine and various vegetable oils contain no cholesterol themselves, all vegetable fats contain some proportion of saturated fat. (Canola oil, considered the healthiest, is 7 percent saturated. Olive oil is 13 percent saturated.) Saturated fat is the building block of the cholesterol manufactured in the liver.

Cholesterol cannot travel on its own accord. It moves through the bloodstream by bonding to two types of one-way vehicles, which are comprised essentially of proteins and called lipoproteins ("lipo" means fat, and cholesterol is a fatlike substance). Low-density lipoproteins, commonly referred to as LDLs or "bad" cholesterol, carry cholesterol and other fats from the liver into the bloodstream, where they are deposited on the artery walls. High-density lipoproteins—HDLs or "good" cholesterol (thinking of HDLs as "healthy" cholesterol helps in distinguishing them from LDLs)—scavenges fat out of the bloodstream and returns it to the liver for excretion from the body. As logic suggests, and most people believe, the fewer LDLs one has and the greater the proportion of HDLs to total cholesterol, the healthier the arteries are likely to be.

Cholesterol in the bloodstream gets back into the liver through "doors" called cholesterol receptors. When the liver holds an ample supply of cholesterol, these receptors close, preventing the HDLs from completing their return trip. A diet high in saturated fat, therefore, contributes to high cholesterol in two ways: by providing enough raw material for the liver to make excessive cholesterol, and, as a result, by closing the cholesterol receptors and trapping the cholesterol in the bloodstream. In contrast, if the liver is low on cholesterol it becomes particularly receptive to the returning HDLs. Thus, a diet low in saturated fats helps to rid the blood of excess cholesterol. In the parlance of blood tests, this translates to high levels of HDL and low levels of LDL.

Government cholesterol recommendations, however, make scant reference to LDL and HDL. Instead, the National Cholesterol Education Program talks about total cholesterol.

The official guidelines, published in 1987, are as follows: Cholesterol levels below 200 milligrams per deciliter (mg/dL) of blood constitute a low risk of heart disease. Readings between 200 and 239 mg/dL are considered "borderline," meaning that people with counts in this range who already have established heart disease or who register two other risk factors are in danger. For those otherwise not threatened, total cholesterol count does not become worrisome unless it runs to 240 or higher.

These guidelines, which predate our present understanding of LDL and HDL, came originally from the Framingham study. According to William Castelli, M.D., current director of the project, one number— 240—jumped off the pages of the Framingham data. This was the average cholesterol count of those who had suffered heart attacks. In addition, Dr. Castelli noted most heart attacks occur in people with cholesterol in the 200 to 240 range, and he has never seen a heart attack in anyone with cholesterol under 150. Furthermore, recent data suggest that for each 1 percent rise in cholesterol, the risk of heart attack increases 2 to 3 percent.

But this cause-and-effect relationship pertained most convincingly to middle-aged men. The Framingham data further suggests that while elevated cholesterol clearly endangered men at high risk, only women in the forty to fifty age group were comparably affected. Even among these women, the association was not as strong as it was in men. It grew weaker with advancing age for both sexes. In the elderly, where coronary heart disease is most prevalent, the correlation disappeared entirely.

Other studies have recently begun to assess how cholesterol affects health, disease, and death in women, the elderly, minority groups, and patients with confirmed coronary heart disease and other illnesses. As these studies come in, evidence is mounting to confirm that high cholesterol does endanger women and that lowering cholesterol helps even people over seventy-five live longer. Still, no one

Estimated Percentage of American Adults with Serum Cholesterol of 240 mg/dL or More

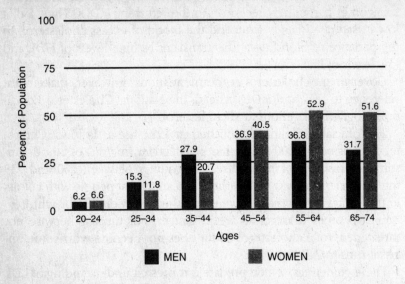

Estimated Percentage of American Adults with Serum Cholesterol of 200 mg/dL or More

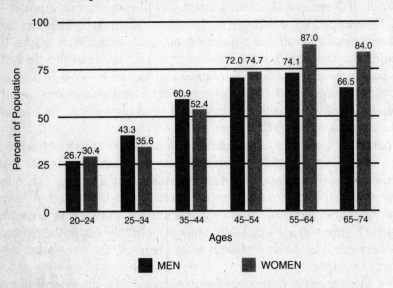

Although young women generally have low cholesterol, by age 54, their cholesterol levels tend to be higher than men's.

Source: National Health and Nutritional Survey, 1976-1980 (NHANES II), National Center for Health Statistics, Reproduced with permission from *1992 Heart and Stroke Facts*, 1991, p. 9. Copyright © American Heart Association, Dallas, Texas.

knows for sure whether maintaining a "desirable" cholesterol of 200 can save women's lives.

Within the past few years, research has begun to tease apart the separate influences of various kinds of cholesterol. In the process, it has become clear that total cholesterol is a crude measure. What has traditionally been communicated as the danger of cholesterol is, more precisely, the danger of high LDL and low HDL. When high total cholesterol reflects a disproportionately high LDL, then high total cholesterol is unhealthy. If, on the other hand, total cholesterol is high because HDL is high, then it is not dangerous. In other words, statistical analyses have finally confirmed what our understanding of the cholesterol mechanism has long implied.

Ideally, we should not be measuring total cholesterol at all, but LDL and HDL separately. And we should be urging women to strive for LDL levels below 130 and HDL levels above 55. But measuring LDL requires a costly test run on a blood sample drawn after twelve to fourteen hours without food. This protocol is too expensive and cumbersome for screening huge numbers of people. Since it is easier to measure total cholesterol and HDL, LDL is commonly evaluated indirectly by looking at what proportion of the total cholesterol HDL occupies. This proportion is expressed as a ratio of total cholesterol to HDL. If your total cholesterol were 200 and your HDL cholesterol were 40, it would be written as a fraction, 200/40, which reduces to 5/1. Expressed as a ratio, this fraction would read 5:1, or, more simply, 5.

This ratio of total cholesterol to HDL is a more precise prediction of risk than total cholesterol—so much so that in February 1992, the National Institutes of Health formally urged all adults having routine cholesterol tests to learn their total cholesterol/HDL ratio. Several studies show that even if their total cholesterol is low, when their HDL is also low, men and women encounter a surprisingly high rate of heart attack. According to the newest research, a ratio of less than 3.5 is desirable. A ratio between 3.5 and 6.9 constitutes moderate risk and anything over 7.0 is clearly dangerous. Thus, the cholesterol profile used in the illustration above is more dangerous than a profile comprised of a total cholesterol of 250 and an HDL of 96 (ratio of 2.6) even though the latter total cholesterol is higher.

The importance of HDL is particularly relevant to women since women characteristically have higher HDLs than men. Their HDLs peak during the childbearing years. Even after menopause, when

HDL tends to fall and total cholesterol rise, women maintain the HDL edge.

This is not to say that high cholesterol does not threaten women. On the contrary, levels rise steeply as women hit middle age. Even if you have always had low cholesterol, it is likely to start creeping up during middle age. By the time they reach age fifty-five, high cholesterol threatens women more than men. The danger is compounded when young women with low cholesterol perceive themselves as invincible and ignore the principles of low-fat eating (which are described in detail in Chapter 10).

In his 1989 book, *Heart Failure*, writer Thomas Moore highlighted a number of critical questions that research had yet to answer. Specifically, at what point does cholesterol really become a problem for people other than middle-aged men? Are the benefits of lowering cholesterol with medication worth the potential side effects and risks? Is it possible to lower cholesterol too much, thereby increasing risk of other diseases? Is it possible to lower cholesterol enough to alter the course of atherosclerosis? While Moore acknowledged that high cholesterol clearly increases risk for some people, he accused the National Cholesterol Education Program of acting irresponsibly by establishing sweeping public health policy without answers to these questions.

Moore's case, which makes some valid points, suffered a serious blow when the most definitive cholesterol study to date was published in October 1990. This was the first study to provide valid statistical proof that lowering cholesterol can prevent nonfatal heart attacks. In this study of 763 men and 75 women—as usual, women were grossly underrepresented—half the patients underwent the most drastic treatment for cholesterol possible: They submitted to abdominal surgery to bypass the part of the small intestine where cholesterol enters the bloodstream. By closing off this part of the small intestine, cholesterol was instead forced into the large intestine and then excreted. After this surgery, patients experienced a 23 percent drop in cholesterol, their counts falling from an average 251 to 196. The other half of patients in the study, who received conventional care, experienced a drop of less than 1 percent.

During the project's ten-year duration, total death rates for the two groups were close. But for those who had no apparent heart disease at the outset of the study, this operation provided noteworthy protection. One third of those in the surgery group avoided fatal heart attacks. The total number of heart attacks, fatal as well as nonfatal, was 35 percent lower in the surgery group, and this group needed fewer than half the coronary bypass operations of the other group. Most significant of all, periodic *angiograms* (X-ray studies that show blockages in the coronary arteries) demonstrated quantitatively that when plaque accumulates at a slower rate, patients tend to have fewer major coronary events.

While this study does not imply that surgery is the best solution to the cholesterol problem, it proved that lowering cholesterol can stave off heart disease. For Antonio Gotto, M.D., chief of medicine at Baylor College of Medicine and former president of the American Heart Association, this study was "the smoking pistol." The University of Chicago's Dr. Paul Meier, who has always felt uncomfortable with the National Cholesterol Education Program's message, said that he was impressed by the angiographic evidence. "It provides some evidence of what has heretofore been strictly theory," he said. Harvard's Dr. Thomas Chalmers, who called this the most impressive study to date, said it persuaded him to begin advising low-fat diets for adults at high risk.

Since this study, other research has shown that it is not only possible to slow atherosclerosis but also to actually turn it around. One of these studies, by Dean Ornish, M.D., showed that this feat could be accomplished solely through changes in diet, exercise, and stress reduction. A second trial, by Linda Cashin-Hamphill, M.D., and associates, achieved similar results by combining a low-fat diet with cholesterol-lowering drugs. Angiographic evidence, combined with patients' reduction in pain and improvement in life-style, confirms that reducing cholesterol can have a significant impact on heart disease.

It's one thing to believe that high cholesterol is dangerous and that lowering it offers some protection. It's another to discover whether you are at risk. Portable analyzers that provide an instant assessment from a finger prick of blood—the kind you might find at shopping malls—are notoriously inaccurate, and the technicians who operate them often are poorly trained. Although the National Cholesterol Education Program urged laboratories to assure that their evaluations fall within 5 percent of true value, only half the laboratories met that standard between 1985 and 1987.

To compound the problem, cholesterol levels naturally rise and fall, sometimes dramatically, with changes in diet, weight, alcohol use, smoking, exercise, and season of the year. In one study of twenty people, four weekly cholesterol measurements revealed swings of more than 20 percent in fifteen of the participants. On a cholesterol count of 200, these variations could result in readings ranging from 180 to 220.

To get the most accurate reading possible, your blood should be analyzed at a laboratory certified by the Lipid Research Clinics, preferably by the same laboratory each time. You will get the most accurate assessment if you have your blood drawn after having eaten nothing for twelve to fourteen hours—a so-called fasting test. If possible, therefore, arrange to have your test before breakfast. To compensate for unavoidable variations, if your reading is high, the National Institutes of Health recommend that you have three tests taken at one-week intervals. This repetition is necessary only if medication is being considered. If your cholesterol is normal and you are under forty, one test every five years is sufficient. If you are over age forty, have the test repeated every year.

Triglycerides, another blood fat, seem to play a role in heart disease, but the exact nature of that role is not clearly understood. Researchers suspect that triglycerides have something to do with heart disease because of their relationship to dietary fat: Triglyceride levels rise in the blood immediately after you eat fatty foods. The Framingham study suggests that triglycerides form an independent risk for women, but not for men. Other research suggests that triglycerides pose an independent heart disease risk for diabetics. And people with heart disease tend to have elevated triglycerides. But triglyceride levels also tend to go hand in hand with low HDL levels. And some researchers have shown that when you statistically eliminate cholesterol, the triglyceride connection becomes weaker. In some instances, the link disappears entirely. In short, while study after study has noted a connection, it is not clear just what that connection is.

Because the relationship between these blood fats and heart disease is fuzzy, experts disagree on what to do about triglycerides. In fact, there are more questions than answers pervading the entire subject: What constitutes normal levels? While normal is generally defined as 30 to 175 milligrams per deciliter of blood, some labs put the upper limit of normal at 150 and others put it at 200. Fasting triglyceride levels between 50 and 250 are considered borderline, and anything above 250 is considered high. But new research suggests that you might be able to get a more accurate sense of how someone metabolizes triglycerides by measuring them immediately after a "standard meal." If so, what constitutes a standard meal, and what should the cutoff points be between normal, borderline, and high? And if triglycerides do in fact play a part in causing heart disease, what are the dynamics of that relationship? Most experts agree that the role is neither as strong nor as direct as that of cholesterol.

While there is no consensus on how high triglycerides can harm you, everyone agrees that low triglycerides are better. If your triglycerides are high, the first step is find out why. Sometimes, genetic abnormalities cause the problem. It is also linked to certain medications—including some diuretics, beta blockers, birth control pills, and other estrogen preparations—as well as diabetes, kidney disease, and obesity. Cutting back on sweets (the culprit is simple sugar), losing weight, and exercising regularly help to control triglycerides. And since alcohol affects the way the body metabolizes fats, avoiding alcoholic beverages may help. Since research has yet to show that lowering triglyceride levels plays a part in the prevention or treatment of heart disease, most experts would not prescribe medication to lower triglycerides unless they exceed 1,000 milligrams per deciliter, at which point these blood fats can cause a painful and potentially dangerous inflammation of the pancreas.

SMOKING

It's no news that cigarette smoking is lethal, and that the longer you smoke the greater your peril. This truth assumed new proportion in April 1992, when it was announced that cigarettes contribute to 25 percent of deaths in the state of Oregon. Three years ago, Oregon became the first state to require death certificates to indicate whether tobacco contributed to the cause of death. Analysis of these records showed that cigarettes caused more premature deaths than automobile accidents, suicides, homicides, and AIDS combined. The victims, who died from breathing disorders, cancer, diabetes, flu, and pneumonia as well as from heart disease, strokes, and other circulatory disorders, included 688 adults who succumbed to the perils of second-hand smoke and 43 infants whose deaths were linked to their mothers' smoking during pregnancy.

Where heart disease is concerned, carbon monoxide, cyanide, formaldehyde, and other poisons absorbed with every puff work together to strain the cardiovascular system. Within seconds, the toxins raise your heart rate by twenty-five beats a minute and blood pressure by twenty points. Carbon monoxide chokes out oxygen in the blood while nicotine shrinks blood vessels and shuts down bypass grafts. In addition, smoking encourages the blood to clot, raises LDL cholesterol, and injures the lining of the arteries. For these reasons, smokers have 70 percent more heart attacks than nonsmokers. Worse, preliminary research has implicated nicotine, which seems to have some capacity to mask pain, as a culprit in silent heart attacks.

The data on women who smoke is incontrovertible. Moreover, younger women, who are otherwise at very low risk, have the highest vulnerability. One of the largest ongoing studies of women, the Harvard Nurses Health Study, which began in 1976 with 120,000 participants aged thirty to fifty-five, documented that smokers succumb to heart attacks five times more than nonsmokers. The Framingham study showed that fifty-five-year-old women who smoke are more vulnerable to fatal heart attacks than men of the same age. And according to a recent study published by the Mayo Clinic, smoking is the single cause in two out of three cases of severe coronary heart disease among women aged forty to fifty-nine. What's more, just a few cigarettes a day do a lot of damage; smoking between one and four cigarettes a day raised heart disease rates nearly two and a half times among the Harvard nurses, claiming responsibility for 58 percent of their disease. Thus Walter Willett, M.D., codirector of the Nurses Health Study, doesn't hesitate to label smoking "far and away" the leading controllable cause of heart disease.

Secondary smoke is nearly as dangerous. One hour in a smoke-filled room is equivalent to smoking one cigarette, the Surgeon General estimated in 1989. After two hours in a poorly ventilated room, the carbon monoxide level in the blood of nonsmokers doubles. In 1990, the EPA concluded that, because side-stream smoke causes 3,800 lung cancer deaths a year, it deserves to be labeled a "class-A carcinogen." And according to research out of San Francisco in 1990, when one spouse in a marriage smokes, the nonsmoker incurs one third more lung cancer and heart disease than mates of nonsmokers. However, because heart disease is ten times more prevalent than lung cancer, the consequences are ten times more profound: an estimated 30,000 to 40,000 deaths a year. One small 1985 study by Elizabeth Barrett-Connor, M.D., and her colleagues at the University of California, San Diego, not conclusive by itself but reliable because its results parallel others, documents a quantitative correlation between the number of cigarettes that a husband smokes and the age at which his wife will die from heart disease.

Women in large numbers did not begin smoking until after World War II and, even then, did not smoke as heavily as men. Since smoking does its damage silently for the first twenty or thirty years, the risks that female smokers incurred did not become apparent until relatively recently. Before World War II, women had sharply lower rates of lung cancer and heart disease than men. Less entrenched smoking habits deserved considerable credit for women's longevity, 78.3 years in 1983 compared to 71 years for men. But in 1985 lung cancer for the first time killed more women aged fifty-five to seventy-four than breast cancer, a clear indication that smoking was taking its toll.

Ironically, because it takes twenty to thirty years for damage from smoking to show up, women had already begun to break the habit before its dirty work appeared. In the twenty years following the Surgeons General's landmark alert in 1964, the number of female smokers declined 12 percent. But the twenty-five million women who continue to smoke are smoking more now than ever before, particularly teenage girls. They account for less than 4 percent of cigarette sales, yet the trend is frightening. Between 1980 and 1983, the number of seventeen- to eighteen-year-old smokers rose 31 percent. For thirteen- to sixteen-year-olds, the rate was 12 percent. The babies took the lead. The number of twelve- to fourteen-year-old girls who smoke tripled during these three years. These statistics take on added significance with the realization that most adult smokers get hooked before they turn twenty. These young women could well become future heart disease statistics.

OBESITY

As a nation, Americans are the fattest people in the world, and we're getting fatter. Half of all black women and a quarter of all white women weigh too much, according to the Metropolitan Life Insurance tables. One in five middle-aged American women is 30 percent overweight, and these women suffer three times the cardiac crises as those who are lean.

As weight climbs farther and farther past ideal, the more coronary artery disease progresses. If you weigh just 10 percent more than normal, you risk a 30 percent higher chance of a heart attack, and if you're 15 to 29 percent overweight, your risk more than doubles. This impressive data, gleaned from the Harvard Nurses Study in 1990, held even after statistical adjustments for smoking, which helps keep weight down.

Yet the available research is incomplete. The Harvard research, whose results jibe with most similar studies, looked only at relative weight, not at weight distribution. Separate studies document that if you carry your excess weight below your waist, you are less vulnerable to heart disease than if your excess gravitates to your middle. These findings, first published in 1956 and confirmed repeatedly thereafter, reveal that women with "love handles" are more vulnerable to high blood pressure, high cholesterol, and diabetes than women with "saddlebags." This correlation is so strong that one researcher suggested studies should compare heart disease in apple-shaped people and pear-shaped people, not men and women. How does weight distribution affect the impact of excess weight? The Harvard research did not address this question.

How does exercise alter the picture? If you are diligent about your sit-ups and flatten your tummy, do you lower your risk? Is weight distribution an indicator of risk by itself, or does it falsely appear to be a risk factor because it is commonly associated with high cholesterol, high blood pressure, diabetes, and other factors? If cause and effect is operative here, which is the cause and which is the effect? How does the relationship of total body weight to percent of body fat influence risk? Since muscle weighs more than fat and the proportion of muscle reflects physical condition, it would seem logical that as weight attributed to muscle increases, risk of heart disease would decrease. Yet research has yet to answer these questions.

While the particular dynamics of excess weight and heart disease still need to be clarified, there is no question that some significant correlation exists. Among women with coronary artery disease, 70 percent are significantly overweight. Obesity often goes hand in hand with high blood pressure, high cholesterol, high triglycerides, and diabetes. Moreover, as weight comes down, these associated risks also diminish.

Problem: Losing weight and keeping it off pose a particular challenge to women. To meet the demands of pregnancy, women's bodies naturally hold a higher fat-to-muscle ratio than men's. And, because women's metabolism is lower than men's, women have a harder time shedding excess pounds and keeping them off. After

1983 METROPOLITAN HEIGHT AND WEIGHT TABLES

		WOMEN		
HEIGHT		SMALL	MEDIUM	LARGE
FEET	INCHES	FRAME	FRAME	FRAME
4	10	102–111	109–121	118–131
4	11	103–113	111–123	120–134
5	0	104–116	113–126	122–137
5	1	106–118	115–129	125–140
5	2	108–121	118–132	128–143
5	3	111–124	121–135	131–147
5	4	114–127	124–138	134–151
5	5	117–130	127–141	137–155
5	6	120–133	130–144	140–159
5	7	123–136	133–147	143–163
5	8	126–139	136–150	146–167
5	9	129–142	139–153	149–170
5	10	132–145	142–156	152–173
5	11	135–148	145–159	155–176
6	0	138–151	148–162	158–179

Source of basic data 1979 Build Study; Society of Actuaries and Association of Life Insurance Medical Directors of America, 1980. Reprinted courtesy of Metropolitan Life Insurance Company.

menopause, when women have a natural tendency to grow heavier, weight control becomes even tougher. To compound the problem, for many American women, exercise is anathema, and although the trend is changing, too many women are sedentary. And they might pay the price with their health.

DIABETES

Diabetes occurs when the body cannot metabolize sugar effectively. Because the pancreas fails to secrete sufficient insulin, excess sugar accumulates in the blood. A number of physiological consequences can result, among them high cholesterol and triglycerides. Over time, uncontrolled diabetes can cause kidney damage, blindness, heart disease, and death.

The disease falls into two categories. In Type I, or insulin-dependent diabetes, the body fails to produce insulin, a hormone that regulates sugar metabolism, and patients must take daily insulin injections to compensate. Once called juvenile diabetes because it usually strikes people younger than thirty, Type I diabetes occurs for no known reason. It does not appear to run in families, and people with the disease are usually thin.

In contrast, Type II occurs when the body produces insulin but, for reasons not well understood, cannot utilize it. Also called adult-onset diabetes, this variety accounts for 90 to 95 percent of all diabetes, the American Diabetes Association estimates, and usually appears after age forty. Ninety percent of these patients are obese, most come from families where the disease is common, and many also have high blood pressure. Often called a woman's disease, Type II diabetes strikes nearly twice the women over forty-five as men the same age. When even mildly obese women are challenged by stress, illness, or surgery, they tend to develop trouble metabolizing sugar, while men do not. This form of the disease can often be prevented, postponed, or controlled by following a prudent diet and achieving desirable body weight. Regular exercise is also important, partly because it promotes weight loss but also because exercise has an insulinlike effect, helping the body to utilize blood sugar more efficiently. Diet, exercise, and weight loss often bring cholesterol and blood pressure levels into the normal range as well.

Unless it is meticulously controlled—by insulin in the case of Type I diabetes or by diet and/or oral medication, to lower blood sugar in Type II diabetes—the disease can damage the tiny arteries called *arterioles* throughout the body, compromising blood flow through these vessels and ultimately jeopardizing the organs they feed. As a result, diabetes can lead to kidney failure, blindness, and the loss of limb due to the development of gangrene. When the heart is sabotaged this way, the deficit is so diffuse it goes unnoticed until the muscle becomes damaged and substantial dysfunction results. Because of its association with high cholesterol, diabetes also tends to accelerate the atherosclerotic process.

Diabetes has made Martha Baker miserable. A black woman who looks younger than her fifty-eight years, Martha was diagnosed with diabetes at age forty-one, and within a few years it had ravaged her body. When she was forty-six, she lost a leg. Three years later, her vision began to fail and she had to retire on disability from her career as a computer programmer. By the time she was fifty-five, she needed bypass surgery.

Diabetes negates the benefits of estrogen in premenopausal women and doubles a woman's risk for coronary heart disease. When compounded by obesity, hypertension, high cholesterol, and high triglycerides, as Type II diabetes usually is, risk of coronary heart disease rises fourfold, exceeding the sum of the associated risk factors. Eighty percent of adults with diabetes die from cardiovascular diseases, most notably heart attacks. And women with diabetes die younger than men with diabetes. For some reason, possibly because of a complex interaction between blood sugar and female hormones, diabetes imperils women excessively. When women with diabetes suffer a heart attack, they are more likely to die than either diabetic men or nondiabetic women. To make matters worse, long-standing poorly controlled diabetes can also cause nerve damage, which mutes the sensation of pain and increases the possibility that heart disease will be silent.

Adult-onset diabetes is often mild enough to inflict its damage insidiously without any symptoms. Thus, the American Diabetes Association estimates that, in addition to the 5.8 million people already diagnosed, an alarming 4 to 5 million are walking around with diabetes and don't know it. If you have close relatives with the disorder or if your babies weighed more than eight pounds at birth, you have reason to be suspicious. Protect yourself by arranging to have a *glucose tolerance test*, in which one or several blood samples are taken after you drink a sweet beverage and evaluated to see how well your body tolerates a surge of sugar. When diabetes is recognized and blood sugar kept within normal limits, complications can be averted. In fact, according to Centers for Disease Control statistics, deaths from heart disease among diabetics dropped 16 percent between 1980 and 1986.

FORMATION OF BLOOD CLOTS

The development of blood clots is one of the primary ingredients of coronary heart disease. In 1968, the Framingham researchers observed that the blood's propensity to clot had an impact on risk. The more viscous the blood, the more slowly it flows and the more quickly it clots, the higher the risk. This quality of the blood can be assessed by measuring the levels of fibrinogen, one of the blood's clotting factors. Normal fibrinogen levels range from 200 to 400 milligrams per deciliter.

Most people with elevated fibrinogen also smoke and have high blood pressure and diabetes. While the earliest analyses suggested that elevated fibrinogen was more dangerous for men than women, later Framingham data showed that women with levels above 334 mg/dL, which qualifies as high-normal, are also susceptible to heart failure, heart attacks, and clot-related diseases of arteries of the arms and legs. The Framingham Study is the only available research on fibrinogen in women, although four other studies are currently assessing the factor in men.

STRESS

For three quarters of the twentieth century, scientists have known that stress is bad. It causes headaches and ulcers, lowers resistance to infection, and sets the stage for heart disease. This phenomenon was first discovered in 1926 by Hans Selye, M.D., Ph.D., who demonstrated that when rats were exposed to stress, the organs of their immune systems shrank, their adrenal glands enlarged, and ulcers developed in their stomachs.

As Selye's initial work was refined, it became clear that stress is not an absolute entity. Rather, it is defined by perception. If a person finds a particular problem, job, or situation distressing, the feeling will prompt physiological stress responses. If, on the other hand, the circumstance prompts a feeling of challenge or stimulation, the negative physiological reactions do not occur.

Feelings of distress alter the biochemical environment in the brain and central nervous system that, in turn, accelerate the production of adrenaline. Surging adrenaline precipitates the classic fight-or-flight response, which produces a rush of strength and energy. To meet the body's increased demand for oxygen, respiration and heart rate increase while blood pressure rises. To keep the muscles in ready repair, LDL cholesterol levels rise as well (see "Gender as Risk," later in this chapter), just as they do when you eat too much meat. This fight-or-flight response is invaluable in the face of danger. If we need a sudden surge of strength and speed to grab a child out of the path of an oncoming car, it's good to know our bodies can comply. But once we've rescued the child and danger is averted, it's equally important for our bodies to relax, for our adrenaline flow to slack off so our blood pressure can subside, and for our heart rate to slow down.

When distress continues unabated—because there is no way to fit a month's work into a week's time; because the boss makes incessant and unreasonable demands; because your husband is pulling you one way, your mother is pulling you another, and you're forever caught in the middle—the very mechanism designed to protect us from danger puts us in jeopardy. Arteries in the heart and elsewhere, which constrict to increase blood pressure during the fight-or-flight response, fail to relax and become predisposed to spasm. Blood pressure remains elevated, injuring the arteries and inviting clots. Cholesterol levels remain elevated, plaque develops at an accelerated rate, and the stage is set for heart disease.

Research reported late in 1991 suggests that people with heart disease also suffer from an abnormality that makes their coronary arteries constrict excessively during stress. Harvard researchers demonstrated this phenomenon with angiography studies of twenty-six men and women. After taking baseline angiographies, the researchers subjected the participants to stress by asking them to count backwards by sevens from a random three-digit number. As stress mounted, those with clogged arteries experienced a 24 percent constriction of their coronary arteries. In contrast, those with healthy arteries experienced only a 9 percent constriction. Moreover, in the patients with healthy arteries, blood flow increased 10 percent, but in those whose arteries were clogged, blood flow decreased by 27 percent. The researchers theorize that people with atherosclerosis cannot produce normal amounts of a natural substance called *endothelium-derived relaxing factor*, which helps to dilate the blood vessels and offset the effects of adrenaline.

Are these people who are more prone to stress so-called "Type A personalities"? The personality profile first emerged in the late 1950s, when two cardiologists, Dr. Meyer Friedman and Dr. Ray Rosenman, noticed that the upholstery on their waiting room chairs was looking shabby. Apparently, the patients were too restless to sit back and wait their turn calmly. Instead, they agitated at the edge of their seats and wore the upholstery out. From this observation came the now-famous theory that ambitious, aggressive, competitive, hostile feelings put people at risk for heart disease.

When the phrase was coined, the pattern was observed only in men. Research soon documented that women, too, were vulnerable, and by the early 1980s, the National Heart, Lung, and Blood Institute formally pronounced the pattern an independent risk factor for women and men.

As women's liberation took hold, doomsayers anticipated that women were asking for trouble by climbing the corporate ladder. They predicted that as women juggled their responsibilities for home and children with additional demands at the office, they would start dropping from heart attacks in mid-life just as their male counterparts always had. The fear was fueled by studies showing that employed mothers, but not fathers, find juggling these responsibilities stressful. Research further documents that employed women experience higher levels of distress than employed men or housewives. But the expected change in heart disease statistics has not occurred.

The apparent reason: Feelings of satisfaction and high levels of self-esteem seem to mitigate stress. Moreover, research now suggests the assertive, competitive facets of the Type A personality are not damaging, especially when they find constructive outlets, such as challenging professional work. As the work of Duke University's Redford Williams demonstrates, only hostility, cynicism, and frustration appear to be pernicious. Dr. Williams has discovered that these emotions raise blood pressure in Type A people higher than in Type B people. After emotional distress, the heart rate takes longer to slow down in Type A people as well.

In the women's work arena, feelings of frustration and hostility arise most frequently in pink-collar jobs. File clerks and factory workers, for example, are especially vulnerable because their work characteristically imposes substantial pressure without opportunity for control. This scenario causes three times the rate of heart disease in women as white-collar work.

Interestingly, according to a *McCall's* magazine survey of 22,000 women designed specifically to assess stress, the number-one complaint of women worldwide is the inability to control the pace of their work. In addition, this survey found no correlation between stress and the amount of housework a woman does. Those who had children at home did not feel guilty about going to work. Nor did pressure on the job necessarily cause negative symptoms. Women with heavy responsibility affirmed feelings of stress but did not experience the headaches, stomachaches, or feelings of anxiety or hostility that accompany distress.

These findings coincide with some enlightening animal research. The Cynomolgus Macaque monkey, a highly socialized order whose physiology closely resembles that of humans, demonstrated a strong association between status and atherosclerosis. Dominant, successful females developed only a quarter as much plaque as their counterparts lower in the pecking order. Subordinate animals also had higher total cholesterol and weaker total-cholesterol-to-HDL ratios than their dominant peers. Statistically, stress stood out as an independent risk for the subordinate females.

According to hormonal analysis of these monkeys, the dominant females ovulated and menstruated normally, but the subordinate females suffered frequent disruptions in ovulation. What's more, the females with the most extensive plaque deposits had no more estrogen in their blood than did females without ovaries—or males! Not surprisingly, the females with advanced atherosclerosis were all low in status. This research suggests that low social status heightens women's susceptibility to heart disease by suppressing their estrogen and thereby eliminating its hormonal protection.

When we experience harmful stress, we may tend to seek relief by drinking too much alcohol and coffee, smoking, and overeating. Thus stress also has the tendency to incite unhealthy behavior. And according to the Framingham data, when other risk factors are present, stress heightens their impact, thereby exponentially increasing vulnerability.

STIMULANTS

Cocaine, including "crack," or "free-base," and "rock," and amphetamines, known among recreational drug users as "uppers," affect the cardiovascular system in the same manner as stress, but in spades. The drugs stimulate the sympathetic nervous system to increase its production of adrenaline. Surging adrenaline causes severe constriction of the arteries, a sharp rise in blood pressure, rapid and irregular heartbeats, and seizures. Heart rate can accelerate by as much as sixty-eight beats a minute. In otherwise healthy, fit people, this overload can cause death in minutes, even to first-time cocaine users. In addition, cocaine can cause the aorta to rupture, the lungs to fill with fluid, the heart muscle and its lining to become inflamed, blood clots to form in the veins, and strokes to occur as the result of hemorrhaging in the brain. More frightening still, although life-threatening complications are not common, they are virtually unpredictable. They appear to have no correlation to dose, length of use, or method of administration. Research published in 1985 estimated that thirty million Americans had tried cocaine and that six million used it regularly. These numbers qualify cocaine use as the newest risk factor for cardiovascular disease. Whenever a young person who is not otherwise at risk has a heart attack, doctors should consider the possibility of cocaine or amphetamine abuse.

SEDENTARY LIFE-STYLE

A sedentary life-style is nearly as dangerous as smoking and having high cholesterol, and it is far more prevalent. In a survey of 28,000 people from thirty-seven states, only 42 percent exercise at least twenty minutes three times a week. According to this poll, lack of exercise is the most common modifiable risk factor of all.

Regular exercise trains the cardiovascular system, reducing the likelihood of catastrophe when the heart is at rest. On balance, then, exercise serves as an antidote to risk. Regular aerobic exercise lowers resting pulse rate and blood pressure. It reduces total cholesterol and improves the ratio of "good" to "bad" cholesterol. It helps prevent and control diabetes and osteoporosis. It boosts dieting efforts by burning additional calories, raising metabolism, and reducing hunger. It decreases the proportion of body fat. It tempers the craving for nicotine and helps you stop smoking. It helps to clear the lungs and passageways of the toxic effects of breathing cigarette smoke in the environment. And it releases stress while improving mood and generates an overall sense of well-being.

Recent studies show exercise to be effective for young and old, healthy and infirm. One study of formerly sedentary people over age fifty-five demonstrated that an hour of aerobic exercise three times a week paid off in mental as well as physical benefits. In addition to developing greater strength and stamina, the participants' memory improved and they became more adept at reasoning and thinking. Because of these salutary effects, two thirds of the participants were still exercising four years after the study ended.

Even if you suffer from congestive heart failure and were formerly advised against exercising, a 1990 study showed that aerobic exercise can improve your stamina and energy. So can weight training, which has been shown to stave off osteoporosis and increase strength among the elderly enough to keep them self-sufficient. (If you have heart disease, exercise only with your doctor's approval and appropriate supervision.)

Exercise is an important part of our program at the Arizona Heart Institute. While we have no statistics for proof, we observe that patients who are physically fit have an edge on recovering from illness and surgery. The speed with which they bounce back suggests that illness and surgery are tantamount to athletic events, and those who are most fit finish first. In contrast, sedentary patients seem to take longer recovering and have a harder time recapturing their former level of strength. These observations imply that, although you will lose strength and energy if you don't keep exercising regularly, to some extent you can save up the benefits of exercise, just as you can save money in the bank, and withdraw them when your need is greatest.

GENDER AS RISK: BIOLOGICAL DIFFERENCES BETWEEN MEN AND WOMEN

Although men and women are biologically similar, recent research suggests that their respective sex hormones are responsible for subtle but significant differences throughout the body. Sex hormones appear in the developing embryo approximately six weeks after conception and immediately influence the way various organs form. While it remains unclear whether the development of female organs is influenced by the presence of estrogen or the absence of testosterone, we do know that in the male embryo, testosterone changes the enzyme dynamics of the liver, where cholesterol will be manufactured and regulated. Testosterone also affects the developing brain. This has been demonstrated in the laboratory, where infusions of this male hormone into lab animals have changed the physical structure of the embryonic brain.

Hormone receptors identified on the brain give new credence to the theory that some behavioral differences have biological origins. Similarly, sex hormone receptors have been located in the skin—perhaps not surprising considering the acne of adolescence, the milky smooth complexion of pregnancy, and the wrinkling that follows menopause. Estrogen receptors exist on bones and help explain the connection between osteoporosis and menopause. And hormones circulating in the blood apparently alter the action of other body chemicals. A case in point is the enzyme *cyclooxygenase*. In the presence of testosterone, this enzyme produces *thromboxane*, which constricts the blood vessels and encourages blood clotting. But in the presence of estrogen, cyclooxygenase dilates the blood vessels and slows clotting.

Animal researchers have also identified sex hormone receptors on the heart and in the smooth muscle cells of the aorta and other major arteries. Although the effect of these hormone receptors is not clearly understood, their presence is consistent with differences in heart disease observed between women and men.

The biological differences between men and women become particularly pronounced at puberty. As testosterone surges, males, who are biologically engineered to meet the demands of primitive life, acquire a greater capacity to carry oxygen and build muscle. This adaptation, which accounts for an approximate 10 percent advantage in their physical performance over women, is necessary for the strength and stamina primitive men needed for hunting, building, and fighting. This same adaptation, however, increases man's vulnerability to heart disease. At puberty, when male musculature increases, LDL cholesterol also rises, and for good reason: Every time a muscle contracts, the membrane around the muscle fiber is depleted, and cholesterol is needed to rebuild it. In primitive times, men were so active that they needed ready cholesterol to repair their muscles, and they efficiently used up the cholesterol circulating in their bloodstream. Thus, heart disease rarely became a problem. The same holds true today for men who meet comparable levels of physical demand. But when men are sedentary and do not use their LDLs to build muscle, this cholesterol remains in the bloodstream, threatening to clog the arteries. In addition, as the explanation of cyclooxygenase above implies, men are designed to heal quickly when they are injured. But the very mechanism that encourages healing can also cause the clot that lodges in a clogged artery and triggers a heart attack. These physiological idiosyncrasies impose such a striking threat to cardiovascular health that male gender alone is a risk factor.

Females, by comparison, are designed to accommodate the demands of pregnancy and the needs of the fetus. As estrogen surges during puberty, women develop fat stores so that they can nourish their developing babies even in times of famine. The fetus, however, cannot metabolize fats and must be nourished with carbohydrates. To protect the baby, the mother must rid her blood of fats, store what she needs, and convert what the fetus needs to carbohydrates. These tasks are accomplished by HDL cholesterol, which is always higher in women than in men and is highest during pregnancy. Whether a woman has ever been pregnant or not, estrogen helps to eliminate fat from the bloodstream, thereby retarding the buildup of debris on the artery walls.

During pregnancy, blood volume rises by 50 percent and heart rate gradually increases over the nine months, pumping a greater quantity of blood through the body's spaghetti-thin arteries. If these vessels were rigid, blood pressure would rise so intolerably that the arteries would rupture. But estrogen increases their elasticity, and they expand to accommodate the changes of pregnancy. In fact, recent research suggests that pregnancy permanently stretches the arteries and, in some small way, may reduce a mother's liability to heart attack later in life.

Regardless of whether a woman has borne a child, estrogen delays the onset of heart disease in most women by about ten years. Moreover, young and middle-aged women who experience high blood pressure and cholesterol levels encounter less heart disease than men of the same age with identical readings. Similarly, animal research demonstrates that male subjects develop atherosclerotic plaque more rapidly than females fed the same high-fat diet. The converse is also true; on a low-fat diet, women apparently have an easier time slowing, halting, and reversing atherosclerosis than men. Moreover, men with advanced atherosclerosis are more likely to suffer heart attacks than women with identical blockages. While our understanding of these phenomena remains skimpy, these observations correlate with the findings that estrogen receptors have been located on the heart and in the arteries, and they imply that estrogen plays a more complex role in coronary artery disease than simply raising HDL, which whisks fat molecules out of the bloodstream.

The protective effect of estrogen disappears abruptly when the ovaries are surgically removed before the age of natural menopause. In women whose ovaries remain intact, estrogen's protection declines gradually beginning around the age of fifty.

While natural estrogen clearly has a protective effect against heart disease, the picture surrounding supplemental hormones is fuzzier. However, evidence is rapidly amassing to support the merits of replacement estrogen for women after menopause (see Chapter 9).

As for birth control pills, prescriptions once contained high levels of estrogen, which caused blood clots and made women more vulnerable to strokes and other clot-related ailments. As researchers learned how to achieve contraceptive effects with lower amounts of estrogen, this risk declined. At present, oral contraceptives pose few risks for most young women. Risk rises slightly with age, but even in older women, birth control pills pose fewer risks than pregnancy. However, if you smoke, your risk of stroke and other ailments is much greater—as much as twenty times greater if you are older than forty-two. According to the Harvard Nurses Health Study, 70 percent of those who run into heart trouble are smokers. Once women go off the pill, their excess risk quickly abates. Charles Hennekens, M.D., one of the primary investigators of this study, believes that birth control pills are generally safe and effective for nonsmokers under forty and smokers under thirty. "But," he clarified, "I believe that it's better for thirty-year-olds who smoke to quit smoking and take the pill, not the other way around."

Birth control pills also contain synthetic progesterone. Formulations with high amounts of progesterone raise LDL and lower HDL cholesterol, and they aggravate diabetes. But when progesterone is low, these problems decrease. According to one study of over one thousand women, when women took either progesterone alone or 30 to 40 micrograms of estrogen with progesterone their LDL cholesterol dropped significantly. (Their triglycerides rose slightly and their ability to metabolize sugar declined a bit, but neither to worrisome levels.) The results of this study parallel others, which show virtually no increase in heart attacks for women on low-estrogen formulation pills. The results are further verified by a study on monkeys, whose autopsies showed that birth control pills retarded atherosclerosis.

Low-dose oral contraceptives also appear to protect against pelvic inflammatory disease and prevent some two thousand cases of uterine cancer a year. In addition, birth control pills inhibit benign ovarian cysts and approximately two thousand cases of ovarian cancer a year. They also protect the breast from fibroadenoma tumors and fibrocystic disease, neither of which is cancerous but which sometimes requires surgery.

The only possible risk of birth control pills still in question is breast cancer, and the final tally has yet to be taken. There may be a slightly increased risk for the few women from families where breast cancer develops before age thirty-five, and if so, an additional two or three women in 100,000 will be stricken. But for the majority of women who develop breast cancer after age fifty, oral contraceptives seem to offer some defense, reducing the incidence by about 30 in 100,000.

All told, oral contraceptives are credited with preventing nearly 50,000 hospitalizations a year. The American College of Obstetrics and Gynecology recently approved birth control pills for healthy women over forty unless they smoke; weigh 30 percent too much; or have diabetes, high cholesterol, a history of breast cancer, or close female relatives under the age of fifty with heart disease. Moreover, the FDA now believes that the benefits of oral contraceptives in healthy non-smoking women over forty may outweigh the risks.

SOCIOECONOMIC STATUS

People who are poor and poorly educated suffer more illness and die earlier than those who are well educated and financially comfortable. Women as a class are poorer than men regardless of age, race, or ethnicity. In 1987, the mean income for women was $11,435, compared to $22,684 for men. For women over sixty-five, mean income was just $9,547, compared to $16,464 for men the same age. Almost three in four elderly Americans living in poverty are women.

Where there is no money, there is no health insurance, and fewer women have health insurance than men. According to a May 1992 report by the Older Women's League, an advocacy organization based in Washington, D.C., only 55 percent of employed women (compared to 72 percent of men) have medical insurance from the time they turn forty-five until age sixty-five, when Medicare kicks in. Women, particularly minority women, tend to work part time or work for small businesses, which often provide no health benefits. Commonly women rely on their spouses' medical insurance and then find themselves without coverage when they are widowed or divorced. Regardless of cause, although women comprise 52 percent of all forty- to sixty-four-year-olds, they pay 62 percent of out-of-pocket medical expenses.

Gender aside, only 58 percent of blacks, 54 percent of Mexican-Americans, and 51 percent of Puerto Ricans have health insurance, compared to 65 percent of whites and 73 percent of Asians. As many as thirty-seven million people nationwide do not have health insurance. Poor medical care is the corollary to no insurance; poor health habits, including diet and exercise, are the corollary to little education. Racism, unemployment or job dissatisfaction, feelings of failure, and the resulting anger and frustration also figure into the equation. These factors have been implicated in the excessive rates of obesity and high blood pressure among black women and undoubtedly play a part among other groups as well.

The consequences of low socioeconomic status are aggravated by the growing awareness of biological differences among people. Researchers know, for example, that women, the elderly, and various ethnic groups all metabolize drugs differently, but their knowledge of how each group metabolizes various drugs is still crude. When limited knowledge compromises treatment, the patient suffers. And most of the patients who fall victim to the impact of inadequate research also suffer disproportionately from low socioeconomic status.

One way or another, poverty contributes to premature death from many illnesses that are easily treated, among them hypertensive and rheumatic heart disease. Of the 121,560 premature deaths in the United states, 80 percent occurred among American blacks, although they comprise only 13 percent of the United States population.

AGE

For the majority of women, heart disease first appears sometime after fifty, the average age of menopause. At this time women lose their natural estrogen protection. Their cholesterol rates tend to climb dramatically. So does their blood pressure. As the impact of risk factors accelerates, the plaque that has amassed gradually over the years begins accumulating at a faster pace. Meanwhile, like the skin and other tissues, blood vessels lose their elasticity, further impeding coronary circulation. Ultimately symptoms appear.

By the time women have their first heart attack, they are about twenty years older than their male counterparts and, as a result, more likely to be suffering from other chronic problems associated with advanced age. In addition, the majority of women over sixty-five are widowed and often lack the emotional support necessary to overcome a medical crisis (see Chapter 8). By the time women have serious heart disease, their health is often compromised by other ailments, which sometimes make treatment more difficult. When they lack essential emotional support as well, their potential for recovery is further threatened.

Aging is unavoidable. If you are concerned about heart disease, it is particularly important to seek prompt attention and to secure an accurate diagnosis and definitive treatment as early as possible.

FAMILY HISTORY

Family history, primarily on our mother's side, plays an enormous part in our fate. When we tabulated the results of our first heart test at the Arizona Heart Institute, 99.6 percent of those who fell into the high-risk category had close relatives with heart disease. Of those who scored medium risk, 90.4 percent had a positive family history, as compared to just 16.9 percent who scored low.

Sixty-nine-year-old Wanda Ferris, who comes from a family cursed by heart disease, is a prime example. Both her parents died of heart attacks, her older sister died twelve years after bypass surgery, and another sister has multiple cardiac problems. Of her three brothers, two have already died of the disease and the third has undergone bypass surgery. Wanda spent her whole life trying to outwit her heritage. She watched her diet, hiked, played tennis, and when she played golf, she walked the course. Petite and peppy, wearing a warm-up suit and expensive cross-trainers, Wanda looks the picture of vitality. But she could not defy her genes. At age sixty-eight, while doing some tricky maneuvers on water skis, she felt the deep dull pain of angina. A medical exam later revealed she had developed heart disease.

Not long ago, we had another powerful illustration of the impact of family history when a new patient to the AHI explained why she came to see us. "There were ten children in our family," this seventy-year-old woman said, "but now there are just two left. The boys got their heart disease earlier. The girls started at seventy."

People with two immediate family members who suffer a heart attack before the age of fifty-five have five to ten times the risk of contracting early disease themselves, compared with people whose family history is less ominous, according to a study of more than 94,000 people in a closely knit Mormon community.

Genes affect our propensity for high blood pressure, obesity, and diabetes. And sometimes they work in powerful yet puzzling ways. Consider this example: Native Americans have an unusually high rate of diabetes and obesity. In most populations, these conditions would set the stage for heart disease. But as a rule the American Indians don't get it. One study concluded that their saving grace was lower total and LDL cholesterols.

Perhaps the most striking illustration of protective genes is a Kansas City woman who boasts HDL levels four to five times above average. She inherited a rare gene that provides three times the normal amount of an essential component of HDL, called *apolipoprotein A-I*. Born into a family where longevity routinely runs into the eighties, nineties, and beyond, she is the only known human being to have inherited two copies of this "Methuselah gene." Researchers at the National Institutes of Health, who hope to isolate this desirable gene, believe that it holds the potential for developing new therapies to improve cholesterol profiles and raise life expectancy.

Because of good genes, some people can live to ninety with cholesterol levels of 450 while others die at an early age with normal readings. Genes also influence how much cholesterol our bodies absorb from the fatty foods we eat, the extent to which cholesterol levels respond to changes in diet, how many cholesterol receptors we have, and how efficiently they work. And genes determine how resistant our arteries are to cholesterol deposits.

INTERACTION OF RISK FACTORS

Cholesterol, in fact, turns out to be the common denominator among most other risk factors. In one way or another, other risk factors alter the balance of LDL and HDL, increasing or decreasing the likelihood that plaque will build up in the arteries. For example, smoking raises LDL and appears to facilitate its ability to lay down plaque. It also seems to shift the distribution of fat off the saddlebags and onto the love handles, where extra weight is associated with higher LDL levels. And smoking has been linked to early menopause, which also affects the cholesterol ratio negatively.

Similarly, obesity, diabetes, and stress all adversely affect cholesterol. Animal studies have demonstrated that stress catalyzes the buildup of plaque, while lowering stress levels brings down LDL.

Exercise, in contrast, raises HDL, as does the presence of estrogen. Estrogen lowers LDL and enhances HDL, the primary reason why women under fifty are protected from heart disease. When women have their ovaries removed prematurely, as happens when they have total hysterectomies, their HDLs drop and their risk of premature heart attack rises sharply. Women who experience natural menopause before the average age of fifty-one are also at a higher risk, and past the average age of menopause, the incidence of heart disease rises steadily. These observations underlie the rationale for replacing lost estrogen with synthetic supplements. Even oral contraceptives fit the pattern. Only prescriptions containing high doses of progesterone, which, like testosterone, raises LDL and lowers HDL, have significantly adverse effects on cholesterol. Parenthetically, characteristic risks of heart disease in men also fit the pattern: The male hormone testosterone correlates to an adverse cholesterol ratio; the male tendency toward high LDLs and low HDLs contributes to their vulnera-

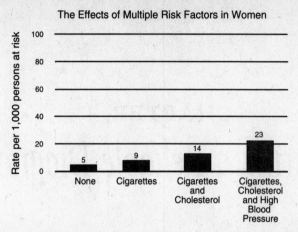

The Effects of Multiple Risk Factors in Women

As the number of risk factors increases, so does the likelihood of having a heart attack. Over a period of eight years, eight in every 1,000 woman (compared to 47 per 1,000 men) will have a heart attack. This chart is based on data from the Framingham Heart Study, Section 37 (August 1987).

Source: Based on charts from *1992 Heart and Stroke Facts*, 1991; published by the American Heart Association, Dallas, Texas, p. 20.

bility to premature heart disease, and because of this correlation male sex stands alone as a risk factor. Clearly, the cholesterol connection to heart disease is consistent and pervasive.

Just as various other risk factors influence cholesterol, so risk factors tend to influence each other. As the number of factors increases, total risk accelerates, sometimes exponentially. Smoking, for example, imposes a statistically greater risk when combined with high blood pressure than with high cholesterol. Similarly, type A personality characteristics are more dangerous in women already susceptible than for those otherwise at low risk.

TAKE ACTION

The good news is, if you reduce your risk, you can often achieve multiple benefits. (A detailed discussion of how to lower your risk appears in Chapter 10.) By reducing your modifiable risks, you can go a long way toward offsetting a genetic predisposition to disease. Even if you've already had a heart attack, you may be able to prevent a second. And if you've never had one, perhaps you never will. With healthy habits and good medical care, you can take charge of most of your risk factors and compensate for the ones you can't control.

CHAPTER 4
Securing a Reliable Diagnosis

One morning, while she was preparing a hunk of clay for the pottery wheel, sixty-two-year-old Bernice Lacey felt an ominous ache in her chest for the first time. She stopped to rest, and the pain faded quickly. Still, Bernice had the good sense to call her doctor. And Bernice's doctor had the good sense to take her symptoms seriously and have Bernice come in for a checkup.

Having looked after Bernice's health for over twenty years, Martin Smith knew her well. Nevertheless, as he and Bernice sat in his private office before her examination, he questioned her intently about her symptoms and their onset. Characteristically, heart disease asserts itself with one or more of the following:

- chest pain and/or pain in the arm, neck, jaw, teeth, and/or back usually but not necessarily associated with physical or emotional exertion
- dizziness, light-headedness, shortness of breath, and/or wheezing
- coughing with or without bringing up blood-tinged mucus

- fatigue and weakness
- swelling of the ankles
- pain in the legs associated with walking and relieved by rest

Dr. Smith was eager to know which of these symptoms Bernice had experienced and how severe each had been. So he probed. "What did your chest pain feel like?" he asked.

"It felt like someone was squeezing my heart," Bernice replied.

"How long did it last?"

"I'd say it was gone within a minute after I sat down."

"And when did you notice it next?"

"I haven't felt it again," Bernice replied, adding that she felt a little foolish for keeping her appointment for symptoms that probably amounted to nothing. "You probably think I'm a hypochondriac, but I just thought I should check this out."

Dr. Smith quickly assured Bernice that her prudence was wise, and he probed further. No, Bernice had no pain anywhere when she walked or exerted herself in other ways. No, her ankles were not swollen, not even after a full day on her feet. No, she was not aware of any palpitations aside from the occasional skips in heartbeat she had experienced all her life. No, she was not coughing or wheezing, and she was certainly not coughing up blood. No, she was not aware of being short of breath.

"What about when you climb stairs? Do you ever notice that by the time you get to the top you're breathing more heavily than you used to?"

"Well, now that you ask . . . About a month ago, I began to notice that when I bring the laundry up from the basement, I have to stop and catch my breath. I figured I'm not as young as I used to be."

Dr. Smith pursued this tack. "Were you out of breath or tired or both?"

"Mostly I just needed to catch my breath. But I do notice I get tired more easily these days. I don't have the energy for evening projects the way I used to. After supper, I'd just rather watch television or get into bed and read."

"Let's go back to feeling short of breath. Do you ever get that feeling when you're walking on level ground? When you carry your groceries in from the car? When you feel upset?"

Bernice didn't think so.

"What about at night? Do you ever feel short of breath while you're lying down? Do you breathe more easily sleeping on an extra pillow?" Again, Bernice said, "No."

Dr. Smith was also interested in Bernice's risk profile. In reviewing her chart, he saw that her blood pressure had been in the high-normal range for years, as had her cholesterol. She did not have diabetes, she was not overweight, and she was taking replacement estrogen; but she exercised only sporadically, and there was a clear pattern of heart disease in her family. Bernice's risk was not pronounced, but it was certainly discernible.

By the time this preliminary interview was over, Dr. Smith had four clues suggesting early heart disease, aside from Bernice's age: a moderate risk profile, one episode of chest pain, some mild shortness of breath, and fatigue. While all of Bernice's symptoms could reflect other conditions as well, Dr. Smith's medical instinct pointed toward heart disease, and when he examined Bernice, he paid particular attention to her cardiovascular system.

"My examination doesn't turn up anything," he told Bernice when he was finished. "But if you've got early stage heart disease, I probably wouldn't see or hear anything, and it does look as though you're healthy in every other respect. The next order of business is for you to have a thorough cardiac workup."

If you have any of the symptoms mentioned in Chapter 2 or the risk factors discussed in Chapter 3, you should also consider seeing your doctor and getting a thorough cardiac workup.

When Dr. Smith referred Bernice to AHI, he gave her some important advice: "Take your husband with you."

In the face of a possibly serious diagnosis, a second pair of ears—a husband's, friend's, or grown child's—can be very valuable. This ally can give you emotional support during your visit and help you remember later exactly what the doctor said. He or she can also help you balance your perceptions and keep your diagnosis in perspective. If possible, take someone who is fluent in the language of medicine, perhaps a friend who is a doctor, dentist, nurse, or medical assistant. Someone comfortable in the medical environment and accustomed to medical jargon is most likely to keep a cool head.

Before your appointment, make a list of the questions you want to ask. When you go, take pen and paper with you to jot down answers to your questions and other points the doctor makes. You might even consider taking a pocket tape recorder to be sure you don't miss anything.

In addition, obtain a copy of all your records and test results from your regular doctor. These are yours; you paid for them and you are entitled to have them. Make sure the cardiologist and any consultants or other specialists you might see in the future also receive copies of your records and tests results, preferably before your appointment so that your visit is as productive—and cost-effective—as possible.

CHOOSING A CARDIOLOGIST

Under most circumstances, you would be referred to a cardiologist by your family physician, as Bernice was. It's conceivable, however, that you might have to find a cardiologist for yourself. Since heart disease is complex, sometimes mysterious, and potentially deadly, you obviously should choose someone who is first-rate: a clinician with solid training, extensive experience, compassion, and good judgment.

To accomplish this goal, look first at basic credentials and choose someone who is board certified. Certification assures that, after medical school and residency, this internist has devoted three years to the intensive study of cardiology and has demonstrated expertise by passing a rigorous set of exams pertaining to the heart, its maladies, and their treatment. Anyone who is board certified earns fellowship in the American College of Cardiology and often uses the letters F.A.C.C. (Fellow of the American College of Cardiology) after the M.D. following his or her name. In addition, it is important to choose someone who graduated from an accredited medical school, took his or her cardiology residency at a medical center with a respected cardiology department, and is currently affiliated with a hospital whose department of cardiology is respected in your community for keeping pace with the latest techniques and technology. If this hospital is also known for the quality of its nursing care and if it has a clinical research and training program, so much the better.

Pertinent data on over 300,000 board-certified medical specialists are published in two multivolume directories available at most public libraries: The Marquis *Directory of Medical Specialists* and the American Board of Medical Specialties' (ABMS) *Compendium of Certified Medical Specialists*. You can also check board certification by phone. Call the American Board of Medical Specialties at 1-800-776-2378. And you can identify physicians who have been disciplined by state or federal governments by checking the *Questionable Doctors* publication, compiled by the Public Citizens Health Research Group and published annually.* Check your local library or contact the Public Citizens Health Research Group at 2000 P Street, N.W., Washington, D.C. 20036 (202-833-3000).

Beyond credentials, a physician's manner and personality make a big difference to some patients. Unfortunately, too many patients select physicians more for their bedside manner than their professional judgment. Sometimes, this practice gets patients into trouble. Ruth Pinna, for example, adored her cardiologist because he was sweet and attentive. But he was ineffective in managing Ruth's disease in spite of his charm and impressive qualifications. Thirty-nine days after Ruth suffered a heart attack, she was still in the ICU because this physician had not been able to stabilize her condition. Her predicament was resolved when she changed physicians.

A physician's availability, professional commitment, and experience in treating other women cannot be summarized in a directory. This is the fiber of personal recommendation. In general, recommendations from other medical professionals are more substantive than those of friends and family. Yet discriminating people without medical training can make reliable referrals. At the same time, while physicians usually refer to colleagues they respect professionally, occasionally they think of their golfing buddies first. In any event, it is important to consider the source of your recommendation and treat the advice accordingly.

Talk to several people and ask them why they suggested this physician. Just because they have gone to him for twenty years or because he untangled a medical mess? Just because she is nice or because she always takes complaints seriously and consistently resolves them effectively? If you ask several people and repeatedly hear the same impressive praise about the same physician, you've probably found someone good.

To many patients, Dr. Mary Grace Warner personifies the ideal. A graduate of the University of Michigan Medical School and former member of the cardiology faculty at Michigan State, Dr. Warner was physician coordinator of cardiac diagnostic testing at Michigan State University Clinical Center before coming to AHI in 1983. Her com-

---

* The number of questionable doctors listed in each edition is part of the publication's title and changes annually. In May 1991, 9,497 *Questionable Doctors* was published. Editors of the 1992 edition anticipated the new number to be upward of 13,000.

petence and concern are clearly evident as soon as she enters the examining room and prepares to question a patient for the first time.

THE CASE OF BERNICE LACEY

By the time Dr. Warner met Bernice, she had already studied the records and test results Dr. Smith had sent to AHI. Dr. Warner would refer to these records for background information and use the test results to avoid unnecessary repetition, but she stopped short of taking Dr. Smith's subjective findings on faith. Despite Dr. Smith's comprehensive notes, Dr. Warner went back over many of the questions he had already asked. Like every good doctor, Dr. Warner knew that the way Bernice answered her questions was as important as the answers themselves, and she wanted all her information firsthand.

"The pain, which you describe as a fist squeezing your heart, would you say it was pressure? Was it dull or was it sharp?"

"Dull, definitely," Bernice responded.

"Did you ever notice pain in your shoulder? Or your left arm? Or your jaw? Or your back?" Dr. Warner asked.

"No, but I did have some shortness of breath and I'm more tired than I used to be," Bernice said. After her interview with Dr. Smith, Bernice was well rehearsed and she gave Dr. Warner a thorough description of her symptoms. It is the patient's job to tell as complete and accurate a story as possible, and Bernice did her part well.

Dr. Warner picked up on Bernice's cues and queried her about the pattern of fatigue and shortness of breath. How long did the episodes last? What brought them on? What eased them? How consistent was the pattern and how often did exceptions occur? To flesh out Bernice's medical history, Dr. Warner asked about medical events that had occurred earlier in Bernice's life, about allergies, ulcers, viruses, and other medical conditions that she had had over the years, about medications she takes regularly. Dr. Warner also reviewed Bernice's risk profile, and at the end of this interview, Dr. Warner had drawn the same preliminary impression as Dr. Smith. Nevertheless, like a good detective, she avoided relying on the clues Dr. Smith had found. Perhaps he had overlooked something. Perhaps he had drawn a false inference. To safeguard against compounding possible errors, Dr. Warner began her assessment from scratch.

As Dr. Warner held the ophthalmoscope up to Bernice's eyes, she commented, "The back of the eye is the one place in the human body where we can see the blood vessels clearly. Sometimes I look into the eyes of patients your age and I see the vessels of an eighty-year-old, but your blood vessels look your age."

Dr. Warner also paid attention to the pulse in Bernice's neck, which yields clues to the function of her heart. Then, as Bernice lay on her side, Dr. Warner studied her chest for visual signs of an abnormal heartbeat. Stethoscope in hand, she listened to Bernice's heart closely as well. Later, when she had methodically worked her way down to Bernice's legs, she firmly pressed her thumb against the skin beneath Bernice's ankle looking for signs of fluid retention, which sometimes occurs when the heart beats inefficiently. If Bernice were retaining fluid, her skin would momentarily show a white imprint where Dr. Warner's thumb had been, but no such fingerprint showed up. Neither did any other clinical findings.

Dr. Warner shared her thinking with Bernice. "Your story sounds like the first symptoms of coronary heart disease, and I think the pain you felt was angina. Your physical examination was unremarkable. That means if you have heart disease, we've caught it early, which is good. We'll run some tests to find out."

Dr. Warner also always makes sure her female patients have routine mammograms and that they have a baseline bone density test to screen for potential osteoporosis. Bernice's record showed she had had both tests.

For the sake of comprehensive diagnosis, virtually all patients at AHI undergo certain preliminary studies, and Bernice was no exception. In addition to routine blood and urine tests, Dr. Warner ordered a resting electrocardiogram (EKG), which traces the electrical activity of the heart, and a chest X ray, which screens for lung tumors and congestion caused by either respiratory or heart disease. By casting the heart in silhouette the chest X ray also shows if the heart is enlarged, another sign of disease, and will provide a view of the spine and permit a crude assessment of Bernice's vulnerability to osteoporosis. While she was at it, Dr. Warner ordered an X ray of Bernice's abdomen to look for an aneurysm of the body's main artery (aorta) which tends to develop just below the kidney. This weak, bubblelike protrusion of artery wall is vulnerable to rupture, and since a ruptured aneurysm is always lethal without emergency treatment, catching it and repairing it before it bursts can be lifesaving. This film would show more of Bernice's spine as well.

Beyond these preliminary tests, the procedure at AHI varies according to what the physician expects to find. Doctors are trained to use the interview and physical examination to arrive at a preliminary diagnosis and then, as economically and efficiently as possible, to use tests to confirm or rule out the diagnosis and to suggest appropriate treatment. If tests disprove their initial theory, they methodically test additional theories in descending order of likelihood.

Believing that Bernice had early coronary heart disease, Dr. Warner set out to confirm this with a gaited exercise, or stress, test, which is designed to bring on angina in susceptible people. If this test confirmed the diagnosis, Bernice would have a cardiac catheterization to assess the extent of her disease and provide essential clues to planning the best treatment. If the stress test was inconclusive, Bernice would have a thallium scan, and if that test confirmed a diagnosis of coronary artery disease, cardiac catheterization would follow.

First, though, Bernice underwent an *echocardiogram* (Figure 4-1). This live-action ultrasound image of the heart is noninvasive and abso-

FIGURE 4-1.

ECHOCARDIOGRAM

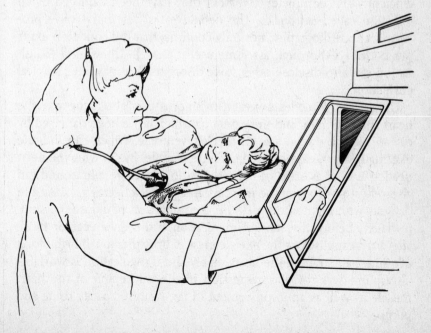

lutely painless. It also provides a wealth of information about the heart. Consequently, it is prescribed for almost every AHI patient early in the diagnostic process. (Bernice's test results and treatment are discussed in Chapter 5.)

ULTRASOUND IMAGING

As Bernice lay on an examining table, the technician coated her chest with a jellylike substance, which would serve as a conductor for the ultrasound wand. Then, as the technician slowly moved this wand, called a *transducer*, across Bernice's chest, a motion picture of her beating heart appeared on the computer monitor beside her. Ultrasound, the same technology used by sailors to read the depth of the ocean floor and by obstetricians to peer into a pregnant uterus, works by sending a sound wave across the chest wall and into the heart. As the waves are reflected, they depict the heart muscle contracting, valves working, and blood rushing through them.

Ultrasound shows the thickness of the heart muscle, the capacity of the chambers to fill, the capability of the pump to contract, and the presence of blood clots. It also shows the status of the valves: whether they are thickened or stiff, whether they open and close efficiently and completely, whether they have been damaged by an infection called *endocarditis*. The definitive test for mitral valve prolapse, echocardiography, not only confirms that the condition exists but permits a thorough assessment of it as well. Ultrasound examination can also disclose other valve disorders that may need surgical correction.

Ultrasound provides a wealth of information about the way the heart is functioning and the extent to which it has been damaged by disease. It shows the size of the left ventricle, which can indicate existing heart disease or predict future trouble. By showing the heart beating as well as areas of muscle that do not move, ultrasound can also reflect portions of the muscle damaged by a heart attack. And in patients with high blood pressure, a comparison of ultrasound studies taken before the start of medication and then a year or more afterward can disclose the effectiveness of drug therapy. If high blood pressure had strained the heart visibly and if medication is working, ultrasound will reveal a regression in the thickening of the heart muscle as well as an improvement of the heart's capacity to fill and pump.

With the addition of Doppler technology, which utilizes the varying lengths of the reflected sound waves, ultrasound can also portray blood flow. Just as you can tell whether a train is coming toward you or going away from you by determining whether the pitch of its whistle rises from low to high or falls from high to low, so Doppler technology interprets the changing length of sound waves reflected by the moving blood to measure its speed and direction. Doppler technology also depicts turbulence caused when inefficient valves permit the blood to churn and swirl back and forth.

Echocardiography is often performed while the patient is at rest, as it was in Bernice's case. If necessary, however, it can be combined with exercise. In such tests, images of the beating heart at rest are compared with images of the beating heart under stress, and differences in motion under these two conditions are analyzed. If this kind of study is needed and the patient cannot exercise because she is ill or disabled, diagnosis can be made by administering a harmless drug such as dipyridamole (Persantine) or adenosine (Adenocard). These drugs quickly dilate the arteries and, when someone has significant blockages in the coronary arteries, cause abnormal contractions of the heart muscle. Ultrasound depicts these abnormal contractions, permitting a diagnosis to be made. In its various forms, echocardiography provides abundant information pertinent to all facets of heart disease, except the status of the coronary arteries themselves.

At AHI we also use ultrasound and Doppler technology to assess the condition of other major arteries throughout the body. Although ultrasound rarely depicts plaque buildup in the coronary arteries because the lungs and other chest structures interrupt the sound waves, ultrasound can show whether plaque deposits are inhibiting blood flow in the carotid arteries, which lead to the brain. Thus, ultrasound of the neck can detect atherosclerotic obstructions that contribute to 75 percent of strokes in our country. As a screening tool, ultrasound imaging of the neck is recommended for anyone who is vulnerable to strokes, specifically people with known coronary artery disease; a history of smoking, high blood pressure, high cholesterol, or diabetes; and everyone over sixty-five.

At AHI, anyone about to undergo invasive management of coronary artery disease has an ultrasound of the neck first because strokes comprise one of the most common complications after heart surgery, balloon angioplasty, and other endovascular procedures. This precaution saves many a patient from disaster, as Audrey Michaelson's story illustrates.

In 1980, when Audrey was fifty-eight, she was diagnosed with exceedingly high blood pressure, which was later fairly well controlled with medication. In 1986, when she complained of a weird swishing sensation in her ears, she had her first ultrasound of the carotid arteries. This test revealed some blockage, but nothing menacing enough to warrant surgical intervention. In 1991, when Audrey needed surgery to repair a knee injury, she returned to AHI for another screening because she knew that atherosclerosis is progressive and that surgery of any kind could trigger a stroke. During the exam, she mentioned that she had had some trouble with her right eye, a problem she attributed to bad glasses. Our workup, however, suggested that her visual disturbance probably came from her carotid blockage. Her carotid ultrasound test showed that her once-minor blockage had progressed and now occluded 90 percent of the right carotid artery. In addition, the test delineated a new narrowing that had developed on the left side. Clearly, orthopedic surgery in the presence of these ominous blockages would have been risky. Although Audrey had never experienced angina, the workup also revealed significant obstructions of three coronary arteries, which would necessitate bypass surgery. Suddenly, Audrey's priorities were reordered and her knee surgery was put on hold.

Since she was most susceptible to stroke, her carotid arteries had to be managed first. She was placed on medication that controlled her heart condition while she underwent an endarterectomy, a procedure to clear the obstructed portion of her carotid artery. After recovering from that operation, she scheduled coronary bypass surgery. Only after recuperating thoroughly would she consider elective surgery on her knee. Although Audrey was forced to continue walking with a cane for more months than she would have preferred, she was saved from a possible stroke by vigilance that began with a checkup and an ultrasound evaluation.

Like most other tests, echocardiography is more reliable in men than in women. In women, breast tissue tends to dull the image. The space between women's ribs tends to be smaller than it is in men, further obscuring the view. If the test is important but ambiguous, an internal ultrasound scan is possible.

In this test, called a transesophageal echocardiogram or TEE for short, a miniature transducer is passed down the throat and into the esophagus. From inside, where neither breast nor bone can interfere, the images emerge vivid and sharp. Unlike a standard echocardiogram, which is easy and absolutely painless, the TEE can be an uncomfortable test. But it is over quickly, and the information it provides makes the brief discomfort worthwhile. A negative TEE saved one recent AHI patient from open-heart surgery after a conventional echocardiogram suggested that a tumor was developing in her heart.

EXERCISE STRESS TESTS

A *gaited exercise test*, commonly called a stress test, is often prescribed to confirm or rule out coronary artery disease. The test makes use of the electrocardiograph, or EKG, to evaluate how well the heart functions while it is subjected to stress. As the patient experiences gradually intensifying cardiac demands, the EKG traces the heart's electrical and rhythmic reactions. Although the test has serious limitations, especially for women, it is inexpensive, and negative results are fairly reliable. In other words, if you're a woman and a stress test says you don't have coronary heart disease, you can trust the report well enough to justify the relatively small cost of the procedure. In men, however, just the reverse is true: A positive test is better than 90 percent reliable, while nearly 40 percent of negative tests are misleading. Thus, stress tests cannot reliably rule out significant coronary artery disease in men.

During the stress test, the patient walks on a treadmill (Figure 4-2). Gradually, the belt picks up speed, forcing her to walk faster. Soon the floor of the machine begins to tilt, making the patient hike up a progressively steeper hill. If the patient develops chest pain or shortness of breath, or if her EKG shows that her heart is struggling to meet her body's increased demand for oxygen, the test is stopped.

Gaited exercise tests are less than perfect for women for several reasons. One, some women who have no heart disease are so unaccustomed to exercising that they do not have the stamina to perform the test. Two, some women suffer from chest pain unrelated to coronary heart disease, and this pain has a tendency to assert itself during stress testing. Three, when women have high blood pressure or an enlarged left ventricle, as older women often do, interpretation of the EKG tracing becomes difficult. Four, women have a prevalence for cardiac idiosyncrasies, such as mitral valve prolapse, which can trigger a false response; although these women do not have coronary heart

EXERCISE STRESS TEST

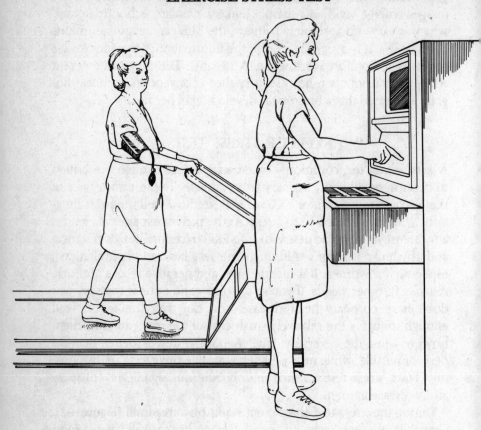

FIGURE 4-2.

disease and may not have chest pain, the stress test tends to trigger an EKG abnormality called a *depressed S-T segment*, which suggests the existence of coronary heart disease.

In one analysis of women's responses on the treadmill, investigators found that 54 percent of women with unrelated chest pain developed symptoms while taking it. In the same study, 38 percent of patients who had no chest pain and who later proved not to have coronary heart disease registered a depressed S-T segment nevertheless. These results led the researchers to comment, "Our data support the premise that in women with 'chest pain' the stress electrocardiogram usually does not add measurably to a secure diagnosis. Certainly, based on these data, a physician would be standing on weak ground in either diagnosing coronary artery disease or ruling it out in a woman with chest pain by considering only the results of a stress test, or more specifically the S-T segment response. Nevertheless, we believe this to be quite common, if not the rule, in general clinical practice."

Because the stress test is inexpensive, researchers have attempted to discover innovative ways to improve it. One strategy utilizes statistical probability to interpret the results and arrive at decisions about further testing. While the goal of this strategy is to make the best possible care available at the lowest possible cost, at least thirteen out of every hundred patients managed this way will slip through the cracks. A more recent and promising approach subjects the EKG reading to complex computerized analysis with a statistical model designed specifically for women. Although the results are impressive, the sophisticated equipment and highly trained personnel required limit the option's availability and increase its cost. Perhaps the best treadmill innovation to date makes use of a simple mathematical formula to evaluate the seriousness of risk on a scale of −15 (low risk) to +25 (high risk). A four-year follow-up of 613 patients evaluated this way showed that the approach could predict survival with 99 percent accuracy. The technique was developed by Duke University researchers and published in the New England Journal of Medicine in September 1991.

In the future, seismocardiography, seismography combined with EKG, may replace stress testing as a screening tool for coronary heart disease. Seismography, well known for its ability to predict earthquakes by measuring vibrations within the earth, can pick up the vibration of the beating heart and measure the pumping activity of the left ventricle. Initial research suggests that, for women, this approach is substantially more accurate than stress testing. Relatively speaking, the test is safe and economical. But additional research is necessary.

THALLIUM SCANS

The thallium exercise scan is a multistep process that incorporates stress testing and a computerized study of the heart to reveal how well or poorly the coronary arteries meet the heart's requirement for oxygen (Figure 4-3). While the stress test demonstrates when blood flow to the heart fails to meet the demand for oxygen, the thallium

THALLIUM SCAN

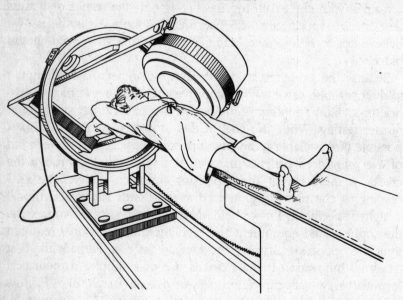

FIGURE 4-3.

test goes a step further to reveal the degree of deprivation. Because its results are also more reliable than those of a standard exercise test, it is often the logical next step in resolving an ambiguous diagnosis.

As the exercise portion of the thallium scan draws to a close, the patient receives an intravenous injection of radioactive thallium. Then, in much the same way that a Geiger counter detects radioactive minerals, a giant scanner tracks the thallium in the blood as it reaches the heart and infiltrates the heart muscle. By picking up signals from the thallium, the scanner can identify where blood has penetrated and where it has not.

For patients whose health or disabilities keep them from exercising, thallium scans, like echocardiography, can be used in conjunction with adenosine or Persantine. These drugs dilate the coronary arteries to mimic the physiologic effect of exercise. This brand-new technology holds great diagnostic promise for the 30 percent of patients, many of them older women, who cannot exercise strenuously enough for a productive exercise test.

While thallium scans are substantially more reliable than simple stress tests, they occasionally imply that disease exists when it does not. In some instances—not well understood but sometimes seen in patients with diabetes or significant high blood pressure—the coronary arteries fail to dilate in response to exercise. Because of this condition, called *endothelium dilating factor* or *coronary artery dilating factor*, the heart muscle receives inadequate blood flow, just as it would if an obstruction were present, and produces comparable EKG tracings. More commonly, in women the breast intervenes between the camera and its target, compromising the clarity of the image in a manner that suggests insufficient blood flow. With these exceptions, thallium scans reliably confirm that coronary heart disease exists and provide valuable information for pinpointing diagnosis.

Occasionally, thallium scans can also miss existing disease. The test is designed to contrast areas of the heart that receive adequate blood flow at the peak of exercise with areas that do not, and if the contrast is not apparent, disease will not be visible. In one such scenario, heart disease could be so diffuse that all areas of the heart muscle are equally deprived. Alternatively, atherosclerosis could be present in a small vessel that supplies too small an area to show up. Nevertheless, the test can, with substantial reliability, rule out coronary heart disease in patients who don't have it. For men, who run a higher rate of false-negative stress tests, a negative thallium scan pretty well rules out heart disease. For women who have a false-positive stress test or unusual symptoms, a negative scan is equally reassuring.

Separate from its use as a screening device, a thallium scan is a valuable aid for planning treatment when coronary artery obstructions exist because the test can also show where previous heart attacks have damaged heart muscle permanently. If an area is hopelessly scarred, it would make no sense to try and improve blood flow to it by angioplasty or bypass surgery. If, on the other hand, the area has never been damaged, angioplasty or bypass might protect it.

PET SCANS: WAVE OF THE FUTURE

Adaptations of *positron emission tomography* (PET) scans hold enormous diagnostic potential to complement thallium scans. This ultrasophisticated computer-assisted test can reveal heart muscle viability at the cellular level. In other words, PET scans document that permanently scarred areas have within them clusters of living cells. Today, PET scans of the heart are experimental and very expensive. As research accumulates and cost diminishes, however, PET scans may some day permit cardiologists to detect vitality in areas of the heart once accepted as dead and devise treatment accordingly.

CARDIAC CATHETERIZATION

Cardiac angiography, commonly but not quite accurately* referred to as cardiac catheterization, is one application of a class of tests (*angiography*) used to assess and plan treatment for the blood vessels of various organs, such as the brain, kidney, legs, and, of course, the heart. In cardiac angiography, the heart and its arteries are visualized using a continuous X-ray beam (*fluoroscopy*) whose image is projected on a monitor. This examination is the ultimate diagnostic test for coronary artery disease. While echocardiography and thallium scanning can imply the existence and extent of disease, only cardiac angiography, an invasive procedure also referred to as an *arteriogram* or dye test, can reveal the condition of the arteries themselves.

The procedure begins when a specially trained invasive cardiologist makes a small opening either in the thigh into the femoral artery or in the arm into the brachial artery. The cardiologist then inserts a catheter and snakes it up to the chest and into the coronary arteries. Once the catheter is properly positioned, a radiopaque dye is introduced to delineate the arteries and the blood circulating through them. As the dye reaches the coronary arteries, which have been all but invisible until now, they suddenly paint themselves onto the X-ray picture of the heart to reveal a veritable road map of circulation. This map clearly depicts any blockages, defining their precise location, scope, and size.

At this point, if the arteries are clear, the cardiologist can test for two other conditions whose symptoms mimic coronary artery disease. To test for variant (Prinzmetal's) angina, that is, angina caused by spasm rather than blockage of the artery, the cardiologist administers a drug called ergonovine, which induces spasm only in people with this condition. If spasm does not occur, the cardiologist can look for syndrome X, a painful but innocuous condition caused by spasms in the microscopic branches of the coronary arteries. Since these tiny

---

* Technically speaking, cardiac catheterization means inserting a slim tube (catheter) into the heart for diagnosis or treatment. Angiography is one of several diagnostic studies possible during catheterization.

vessels are too small to show up on the angiogram, the disorder is usually not visible, but its consequences can be verified by analyzing samples of blood drawn during catheterization. When blood taken from the veins leading out of the heart reveals that areas of the heart have received insufficient oxygen, microvascular spasm is deemed the cause. (For more on Prinzmetal's angina and syndrome X, see Chapter 7.)

In addition to confirming all these dynamics of the coronary arteries, angiography also images the mechanical functioning of the heart and permits an appraisal of the organ's pumping capability. The comprehensive information derived from this study is critical to determining proper treatment for the patient and precedes coronary angioplasty or heart surgery of any kind.

At most hospitals, angiography is a day-long event. Commonly, patients are admitted early in the morning, shaved and prepped as if for surgery, sedated, and wheeled on a stretcher into the "cath lab." During most of these procedures, the catheter is introduced through a puncture in the the femoral artery, which has been numbed by local anesthetic. After the procedure the catheter is removed and prolonged pressure is applied to the wound so that there will be no bleeding at the puncture site. Patients then lie still for some eight hours, until the clot has formed. Often they are hospitalized overnight.

At AHI, catheterization takes on a less imposing feel. Patients generally have no need for sedation and walk into the cath lab unassisted. Instead of gaining access through the femoral artery, which requires hours of immobility after the procedure, the AHI specialists prefer to go in through the brachial artery in the arm. This artery can be opened with a surgical incision and, at the end of the procedure, stitched closed and bandaged in such a way that patients can get up and move about as soon as the procedure is finished. The catheterization, which is done under local anesthetic, takes about an hour. To make sure that no complications set in, patients spend an hour or so in a recovery area, where their families can be with them. Then, after going over the results with the cardiologist, they can go home. Although the brachial approach requires greater technical ability to guide the catheter to the heart, in expert hands, this approach is every bit as safe as the femoral.

When skillfully performed, cardiac catheterization is usually harmless and virtually painless. There is a momentary needle stick when the arm or groin is numbed with local anesthesia. Since the insides of the arteries have no nerve endings, passing the catheter to the heart causes no sensation. Introducing the dye usually triggers a hot flush, and sometimes an unpleasant fishy taste, urgent sense of nausea, and, occasionally vomiting. But in the vast majority of cases, patients do not find the experience traumatic; some even find it intriguing.

Yet there is nothing trivial about it. Technically, it is an exquisitely delicate procedure that results in serious complications in about one in one thousand cases. And for many patients the prospect is terrifying. Some are put off by the consent form, which lists in onerous detail the remote chance of death, heart attack, stroke, or other hazard. Some worry about pain. And some find the notion of touching and imaging the heart an unbearable violation of the soul.

The cost—upward of $5,000—also gives pause, especially in view of the landmark Coronary Artery Surgery Study (CASS registry, 1981–82), documenting that fully half the women subjected to the procedure (compared to 17 percent of the men) did not have significant coronary artery disease. These data, which imply that women were referred for catheterization frivolously, combined with the cost and other potential liabilities, suggest that future recommendations need to be governed by greater prudence and restraint.

However, catheterization is sometimes the only way to rule out coronary artery disease. Although echocardiography, chest X rays, exercise stress tests, and thallium scans overlap somewhat and partially verify each other, separately and together they are imperfect, especially for women. At best, astute diagnostic strategies and careful preliminary tests can minimize the number of patients who undergo catheterization. But until noninvasive testing is improved, cardiac catheterization is bound to be prescribed for some people who do not have heart disease, especially when the patients are women.

Mary McLaughlin is a case in point. She was referred to AHI when she complained of numbness in her hands and pains in her heart. Dr. Warner examined Mary and found a somewhat confusing picture. Her risk profile was suspicious. At age fifty-one, Mary had mild diabetes and slightly elevated blood pressure. Her mother had died suddenly from a heart attack at age sixty-five. Mary's chest pain was sometimes brought on by physical exertion and sometimes by emotional stress, but most often it came with cold weather. Her echocardiogram was normal; her exercise stress test was not, and neither was her thallium scan. Yet Mary's catheterization showed her heart was healthy. She subsequently underwent tests for gallstones, hiatal hernia, and spasm of the esophagus, all of which produce symptoms similar to angina, and she was diagnosed as having hiatal hernia.

Was Dr. Warner wrong in sending Mary for cardiac catheterization? How could any responsible physician have done otherwise? Here was a woman with a history of chest pain, inconclusive tests, and an ominous risk profile punctuated by diabetes, high blood pressure, and a mother who dropped dead at age sixty-five. The possibility of overlooking Mary's heart disease was unthinkable. Besides, confirmation of Mary's clear arteries saved her from the angst that commonly accompanies a diagnosis of heart disease and freed her to live a normal life.

Future developments in noninvasive testing may well save patients like Mary from unnecessary cardiac catheterization. Currently, researchers are trying to adapt *magnetic resonance imaging* (MRI) to screen for coronary artery disease. More promising is the latest generation of CT scanners, call the *ultrafast computerized tomography*. Apparently, this technology, which is currently under clinical investigation, has the unique capability of detecting and quantifying calcification of coronary artery plaque. Since a correlation exists between calcium in the coronary arteries and the development of ischemic heart disease, this noninvasive test, which takes less than ten minutes and exposes patients to about as much radiation as an X ray of the abdomen, may become a reliable screening device, especially for patients under sixty. These innovations remain in the future, however. At present we must rely on cardiac catheterization.

The most compelling reason to pursue catheterization aggressively is the frightful fact that one third of heart attacks go unrecognized and untreated. As discussed in Chapter 2, plaque can develop insidiously and impede blood flow substantially enough to inflict tiny injury after tiny injury upon the heart muscle. Ultimately a massive heart attack occurs and sometimes sudden death. The threat of silent heart disease compels anyone with even the vaguest symptoms to seek medical attention. Anyone whose score on the heart test in Chapter 3 is 33 or above should have regular checkups, during which coronary artery disease can be spotted. Ultimately, diagnosis and strategies for averting disaster rest with catheterization.

Whether your heart disease is silent or screams for attention, unless you have a cardiac catheterization, you and your cardiologist cannot even contemplate angioplasty or surgery. Consequently, unless you pursue catheterization aggressively, you may miss the best time for intervention and set yourself up for trouble later.

In the past, women have not enjoyed the same degree of success from bypass surgery and angioplasty as men. The reason, some studies suggest, is that by the time women receive these interventions, they are older, sicker, and consequently at greater risk than their male counterparts. Separate research affirms that when anyone—male or female—has elective surgery, the results are likely to be better than from emergency surgery. Furthermore, patients who are free of high blood pressure, diabetes, or other chronic disabilities of advanced age also have a leg up. These well-documented assertions support the case for encouraging women to have cardiac catheterization early enough for them to have any necessary invasive management at the optimal time: when their medical condition is advanced enough to warrant intervention but before it deteriorates enough to exacerbate their risk. (For further discussion of this issue, see the section entitled "Bypass Surgery" in Chapter 5.)

THE CASE OF JO-ELLEN WALTERS

Slim, almost frail looking, forty-one-year-old Jo-Ellen Walters came to AHI because of a fainting spell. One morning, shortly after she began her daily routine on her exercise bike, she started feeling dizzy and light-headed. She stopped pedaling and waited for the sensation to fade, but it didn't. When she stood up, Jo-Ellen passed out.

Dr. Warner began to question her closely about the fainting and dizziness. In the process, she learned that although Jo-Ellen had felt faint, she had never passed out before. Yes, sometimes she felt light-headed, especially when she stood up quickly. Yes, sometimes she felt short of breath and found herself struggling to fill her lungs with air. But she didn't have pain in her chest or arm or jaw or back. She had no real pain at all. The closest Jo-Ellen came to pain was a sensation she described as an unusually strong heartbeat, and she had had it since childhood.

"I could sit here and talk to you and feel my heart pounding," she said. By the time she was a young adult, she periodically felt as though her heart were skipping. Then lately, two or three times a day, her body had begun to throb with reverberations.

"Pretty scary, huh," Dr. Warner acknowledged, and Jo-Ellen smiled tentatively for the first time.

Next, Dr. Warner queried Jo-Ellen about her risk profile. Her uncle had died of a heart attack, but no one else in her family had heart disease. Jo-Ellen did not smoke or drink coffee. Her weight, blood pressure, and cholesterol were normal. And she was still getting her period regularly.

"It doesn't sound like coronary heart disease," Dr. Warner said. "You're young, and although women your age occasionally have it, neither your symptom pattern nor your risk profile indicates it. I'm inclined to think we're dealing with mitral valve prolapse."

After examining Jo-Ellen, Dr. Warner was convinced she was on the right track. "You know, I hear a click in there that's consistent with mitral valve prolapse, but we'll do a test to look at the valve more closely. I know that the sensations you've been having are frightening, especially the fainting, but believe it or not, I don't think it's serious. The test will tell us for sure, and if I'm right, we can give you some medication to control your heartbeat. I'm pretty sure we can make you feel better."

While she could almost make the diagnosis just on the basis of Jo-Ellen's medical history and physical examination, Dr. Warner didn't dare. In her more than twenty years as a cardiologist, she has seen many exceptions to many rules, and she doesn't feel comfortable accepting her presumption on faith. So she planned a thorough but conservative evaluation to confirm her diagnosis. Like every good diagnostic strategy, this one was methodical and as prudent, efficient, and economical as possible.

Reviewing Jo-Ellen's record, Dr. Warner saw she had never had a mammogram or a baseline bone density scan, both of which Dr. Warner feels are important for women of this age.

"You should be having mammograms at least every other year during your forties," Dr. Warner advised. "I also think it's important for all women to know their bone density at this time. We're finding that even fertile women in their late twenties and thirties can have low estrogen levels. Inadequate estrogen can lead to bone loss, and if you find out early that you are prone to osteoporosis, there's time to prevent it."

In addition, she scheduled Jo-Ellen for the routine blood and urine tests, chest X ray, and resting EKG. The only other diagnostic test she recommended was an echocardiogram, which provides definitive evaluation of mitral valve prolapse. If Jo-Ellen was in fact suffering from this disorder, the echocardiogram would not only confirm the condition but also permit a full assessment of it. In the unlikely event that she had heart disease of another kind, the echocardiogram would yield important clues.

Jo-Ellen's echocardiogram confirmed that she was suffering from a moderately severe mitral valve prolapse. It further revealed that her mitral valve, though flapping in a manner characteristic of this condition, was working normally and that her heart was pumping effectively. The Doppler study showed her blood to be flowing efficiently. Thus, the echocardiogram confirmed that Jo-Ellen's condition was not severe enough to jeopardize her heart or endanger her health. Since the condition disrupted Jo-Ellen's life considerably, Dr. Warner considered prescribing medication to control her symptoms. (For further discussion of mitral valve prolapse, see Chapter 7.)

THE CASE OF SAUNDRA FELLS

Like Jo-Ellen Walters, Saundra is forty-one years old, but she presents a very different profile. When she was pregnant fifteen and ten years earlier, she had borderline diabetes and very high blood pressure, both of which disappeared after her babies were born. She is thin, and her cholesterol is low, but she had smoked a pack and a half of cigarettes a day before quitting two years earlier. What's more, her father had died suddenly at age forty-seven from a massive heart attack.

Also like Jo-Ellen, Saundra complained of chest discomfort that didn't quite fit the description of coronary heart disease. But it didn't sound like mitral valve prolapse either.

Saundra had had shooting dull pains in the left side of her chest a year earlier, which turned out to be a spasm of her esophagus. Since then, she had continued to feel a different kind of soreness in the upper left part of her chest that seemed to come and go with no apparent pattern. In addition, her husband recently lost his job, her mother had been ill, and her teenage son had been having trouble in school.

After Dr. Warner examined her and found everything normal, Saundra asked, "Could this be anxiety?"

"Maybe," Dr. Warner responded. "But we've got to check it out."

Dr. Warner scheduled Saundra for the same tests she had ordered for Jo-Ellen. When all these tests turned out to be negative, she could almost rule out heart disease. However, because Saundra's symptoms, physical examination, and medical history were equivocal, Dr. Warner also ordered an exercise stress test to make sure she did not have coronary artery disease. Saundra had no trouble on the treadmill. When she tolerated the procedure at its most demanding point, she demonstrated fairly conclusively that she did not have coronary heart disease.

When Saundra met with Dr. Warner to go over her test results, Dr. Warner summed up her findings. "My examination and all the tests we did suggest that you are a very healthy woman. Your chest X ray and echocardiogram were perfectly normal, and you passed the exercise stress test with flying colors. I don't often presume that stress is at issue, but I don't see anything else suspicious here. If you feel that anxiety could be the problem, I'll refer you to someone who can help you manage that. Then, if the symptoms don't go away, we'll have to search more thoroughly for another cause."

Saundra felt comfortable with the plan. "Maybe just knowing I don't have heart disease will let me to relax and I'll feel better."

THE CASE OF HELEN DAVID

"The pain is in my left arm," the sixty-four-year-old widow told Dr. Warner. "When it comes, and that's mostly when I'm in bed at night, it hurts so bad I can't close my hand."

"The pain comes only at night?" Dr. Warner said.

"My hands get numb after work. But the pain comes after I'm in bed and I've been lying down awhile," Helen responded, adding that she works in a laundry and often lifts heavy bundles.

"Do you get numbness in both hands?"

"Yes, but the left is worse."

"You get some numbness in the right hand, though. Do you ever get pain in the right arm?"

"Yeah, but it's worse in the left arm."

"Do you notice any weakness?"

"Well, my arms are not weak, but my legs seem weaker than they used to be."

As Dr. Warner queried further, Helen said she had no problem with shaking, no pain during or immediately after she hauled her bundles, no chest pain, no shortness of breath, no tightness in her chest, no heaviness in her chest or lump in her throat.

Dr. Warner found no other symptoms to suggest that Helen had coronary heart disease. Moreover, she discovered that Helen's risk profile was minimal, her only significant risk factor being the premature loss of her ovaries as the result of a total hysterectomy at age forty-seven. But Helen's cholesterol, which can rise in the absence of estrogen, was only 187. So the hysterectomy seemed to be of minor importance. Her sister had diabetes, but there was no trace of coronary heart disease in Helen's family.

The only other pertinent finding to emerge from Helen's examination was a slight heart murmur, the sound of blood moving somewhat inefficiently through the valves. Like most heart murmurs, Helen's sounded benign.

Yet heart disease is a real possibility in a sixty-four-year-old woman. Moreover, the disease in women is often marked by uncharacteristic symptoms, and the complaint that had brought Helen to AHI could have been atypical angina, which can occur at rest and which is therefore indicative of advanced coronary heart disease. Dr. Warner ordered the same screening tests that she had for Saundra.

"In addition," Dr. Warner told Helen, "I want to test your symptoms with nitroglycerin. I'm going to give you some tablets, and I want you to put one under your tongue whenever you feel the pain in your arm."

Nitroglycerin, the primary ingredient in dynamite, has been used in minute quantities for decades to dilate the coronary arteries. In therapeutic amounts it produces as its worst side effects a short-lived headache and a brief drop in blood pressure. The drop in blood pressure is not dangerous so long as patients take their first dose sitting down, in case they become dizzy or feel faint. Since the drug is safe, Dr. Warner felt comfortable prescribing it as a test. She expected that Helen would find no correlation between taking the tablet and experiencing relief. If, however, Helen discovered that the nitroglycerin helped her pain, she might, in fact, have a covert case of coronary heart disease.

Helen's echocardiogram confirmed that she had a slight mitral valve prolapse that was causing the murmur but that was not threatening her in any way. The nitroglycerin did nothing to ease Helen's pain, and all her other studies were normal, except her exercise stress test.

Before she began the test, Helen's blood pressure was 130/70, well within the normal range. When Helen exercised on the treadmill, however, her systolic blood pressure, which normally should rise to a maximum of 190, went up to 210. And her diastolic blood pressure, which should drop or remain constant, also rose twenty points. This response suggests that Helen's heart's ability to relax is not as good as it should be and that she probably has a tendency toward high blood pressure. In addition, the tracing of her heart showed a depressed S-T segment.

Responding to Helen's look of alarm when she heard this report, Dr. Warner hastened to reassure her. "Everything points to a false positive, and I'm really not worried. But I'll feel better if we know for sure. Just to make certain you don't have heart disease, I want you to have a thallium scan."

As Dr. Warner had suspected, Helen's scan showed that her coronary circulation was good. By verifying that blood flow adequately penetrated Helen's heart muscle even under stress, the thallium scan confirmed the healthy status of her coronary arteries. On the basis of this test, Dr. Warner concluded that the problem in Helen's hands was neurological and referred her to a neurologist for follow-up.

THE CASE OF JOANNE BARNETT

On New Year's Day, just before she turned fifty, Joanne wondered if she was having a heart attack. The pain certainly wasn't classic, but it was awfully suspicious. A sharp, hot pain stabbed her between her breasts and traveled up into her armpit. She thought she would vomit. Stupidly, she refused to let her family call the paramedics, insisting they help her to bed instead. Her husband had some nitroglycerin tablets for chest pain of his own; he gave her one, and she got relief. The next day she saw her doctor, who thought she might have had a heart attack and referred her to a cardiologist, who treated her with medication. By the time Joanne came to AHI, five weeks had elapsed, her pain had grown more insistent, and she had begun experiencing some occasional though frightening palpitations.

Joanne's symptoms, her response to nitroglycerin, and her risk profile all pointed to heart disease. If she had had a heart attack, it would have altered Joanne's resting EKG permanently, but Joanne's study was normal. So was her exercise stress test.

Dr. Warner reviewed the inconclusive evidence with Joanne: "I think we're dealing with variant angina here. [Variant angina is also called Prinzmetal's angina.] If we are, your pain is coming from spasms that periodically squeeze your arteries shut and keep the blood from reaching your heart. The pain you feel is your heart crying out for nourishment, just as it is would if plaque were holding back the blood flow. But if variant angina is in fact the problem, your coronary arteries are likely to be clear. We'll find out for sure when we do a catheterization and look at those arteries. First, though, I want to check out your palpitations and see if we're dealing with a serious rhythm disturbance."

So Dr. Warner had Joanne rigged to a miniature EKG machine, which she wore on a belt around her waist. For twenty-four hours, as Joanne went about her daily business, this Holter monitor recorded her heart's behavior continuously. Joanne also kept a log of her activities so that when Dr. Warner reviewed the EKG tape, she would be able to make sense out of the record by correlating any abnormal tracings to Joanne's activities.

Twice on the day she wore the monitor, Joanne felt the disconcerting throbbing of arrhythmia, but her tracings were within the normal limits and Dr. Warner concluded the palpitations were not serious. The next step was cardiac catheterization, which would reveal the status of her coronary arteries. When the test showed that her arteries were clear, the specialist performing the procedure injected a drug called ergonovine, and a spasm set in right on cue. Once the diagnosis was confirmed, Dr. Warner prescribed medication to keep the condition in check. (For more on Prinzmetal's angina, see Chapter 7.)

THE ART OF DIAGNOSIS

Despite the logic and the appearance of a diagnostic method, the practice of medicine is an art as well as a science, and an imperfect science at that. Consequently, as a good physician takes a patient's history and performs the physical examination, he or she will vary the follow-up studies recommended based on findings and instinct. Art plus science equals judgment. Ultimately, judgment boils down to being thorough without being excessive. And ultimately you must be the one to decide if your physician's judgment is good.

If you question your physician's judgment—because she didn't seem to take your complaints seriously, because her evaluation seemed cursory, because you feel she ordered too many or too few tests, or because the treatment she prescribed didn't make you feel better—get another opinion. Heart disease is serious and the consequences of ineffective care can be grave; protect yourself by seeing another expert. At the very least, having your first physician's findings

TESTS FOR HEART DISEASE

SUSPECTED DIAGNOSIS	SUGGESTED TESTS	AND POSSIBLY
heart disease of any kind	complete blood count, including total and HDL cholesterol; urinalysis; resting EKG; chest X ray; abdominal X ray; echocardiogram	ultrasound of carotid arteries; exercise stress test; cardiac catheterization
coronary heart disease	all preliminary tests plus gaited exercise test or, for women who cannot exercise, artery dilation test using adenosine or Persantine	thallium exercise scan; cardiac catheterization
mitral valve prolapse	all preliminary tests	TEE
other valve disease	all preliminary tests	cardiac catheterization; TEE
variant angina	all preliminary tests	Holter monitor EKG; cardiac catheterization with ergonovine
syndrome X	all preliminary tests plus cardiac catheteritzation with special blood studies	
arrhythmias	all preliminary tests	Holter monitor EKG
heart failure	all preliminary tests	any or all of other tests depending on suspected cause

and recommendations verified will give you peace of mind. At most, it can save you from disaster.

Many people are reluctant to get a second opinion for fear of offending their doctors. The truth is, most physicians welcome the idea. Patients also worry about the expense. Under some circumstances, health insurance covers consultations. In any case, you can minimize cost—as well as time, inconvenience, and discomfort—by making sure that the consulting physician receives a complete copy of your medical records, including lab reports and test results. For diagnostic purposes, the consulting physician can even read your cardiac catheterization films, saving you from having to undergo the test a second time. (For more on second opinions, see Chapters 5 and 8.)

TAKE ACTION

It is no easy job for someone without medical training to evaluate medical care. The job becomes even more difficult when your objectivity is sabotaged by the emotions that can accompany the suspicion or reality of heart disease. If you take your husband, friend, or another advocate with you to your doctor appointment, this person can help you appraise your care. Whether you take an ally or go alone, here are some guidelines for evaluation:

- Good diagnosis begins with a thorough medical history. It is your physician's job to ask enough questions to get a complete picture. Is your physician asking? Listening? And taking you seriously?
- A good diagnosis also depends on a physical examination that starts from scratch. Is your cardiologist approaching your problem presuming that a referring physician already did some of the work, or is she evaluating you without any presumptions about what's wrong?
- Doctors are trained to look first for what they expect to find. Is your physician approaching testing in an economical and efficient manner? If he doesn't find what he expected to find, does he have a sound and thorough strategy for testing additional theories in descending order of likelihood? Is he pursuing his investigation until he arrives at a well-founded conclusion?
- If coronary heart disease is at issue, is your physician contemplating cardiac catheterization? If not, does she have a reason that sounds legitimate? If you're not sure, perhaps you should

get another opinion. (Strategies for assuring that you get good care are further discussed in Chapter 8.)

- Medical research convincingly demonstrates that heart disease can be stalled, slowed, and possibly reversed when patients lower their risks substantially. Is your physician concerned with your risk profile? Did he ask about your diet and exercise patterns? Did he ask whether you smoke and, if you do, is he supportive of your efforts to quit? How strongly does he feel about controlling heart disease by reducing risk?
- The acid test, of course, comes when your physician makes a diagnosis and prescribes treatment. Do you feel better?

If your physician respects you, evaluates your symptoms thoroughly, and prescribes effective treatment, you will know it. You will feel better physically, and you will experience a sound sense of confidence in your physician and yourself.

CHAPTER 5

How to Prevent a Heart Attack If You Have Coronary Heart Disease

The most encouraging feature of heart disease in women is its tendency to develop gradually. By diagnosing and treating the disease early, we have a good chance to stop it before a heart attack ever strikes.

We can accomplish this goal with medication, bypass surgery, and/or angioplasty, all of which go hand in glove with steps designed to reduce risk (see Chapter 10). Although each kind of treatment works differently, in its own way, each compensates for blockages in the coronary arteries and thus keeps the heart muscle supplied with enough blood (and the oxygen that the blood transports) to meet the heart's needs for nourishment. Medications do this by dilating the arteries, as well as by reducing the work of the heart. Bypass surgery accomplishes the same goal by diverting the blood flow around the obstruction, just as detours on roads permit traffic to bypass construction sites.

In angioplasty, which utilizes balloons, lasers, and a variety of miniature cutting devices inside the arteries themselves, the plaque is flattened against the artery wall or removed. Either way, angioplasty widens the channel and restores free blood flow. Each approach to treating heart disease has merits and limitations. The trick is to balance benefit against risk and choose the best treatment or combination of treatments in any given circumstance.

As you'll see at the end of this chapter, there is also evidence that making life-style changes alone—changing the way you eat, exercise, and handle stress—can help prevent and sometimes even reverse heart disease without drugs or surgery.

DRUG THERAPY

Dr. Warner faced just this challenge when she reviewed the diagnostic data on Bernice Lacey, the sixty-two-year-old potter whose brief bout of angina was described in Chapter 4. Although Bernice's ultrasound and chest X ray were normal, about five minutes into her exercise stress test, she felt the fist squeezing her heart for the second time, and the test was stopped. However, her EKG reading was ambiguous, so Bernice was scheduled for a thallium scan. This test disclosed that, when Bernice exercised strenuously, a small area on the back of her heart wasn't getting enough blood. The next day, a cardiac catheterization outlined several long, thin, relatively flat deposits of plaque in two of her coronary arteries. None of them looked terribly menacing, although one protrusion closed off half of her right coronary artery. Since this artery fed the area of her heart that, according to her thallium scan, received inadequate nourishment, it was undoubtedly the source of her pain.

Because Bernice had undergone a thorough, methodical workup, Dr. Warner could feel confident that Bernice's diagnosis was accurate and precise: coronary heart disease in its earliest stages. Fortunately for Bernice, her disease was diagnosed before she had a heart attack. With medical treatment, regular checkups, and a reduction in her risk factors, she might never have one. Preventing a heart attack is the primary benefit and ultimate goal of early diagnosis and intervention.

For Bernice, drug therapy, together with an aggressive program to reduce her risk, was clearly the treatment of choice. Because her blockages were slight, medication would sustain adequate circulation to her heart muscle and keep her from pain. Drug therapy is also desirable when plaque accumulation is too widespread to treat completely with surgery or angioplasty or when the heart and its coronary arteries are small, as they tend to be in small people, most of whom are women. If you've ever tried to thread a needle with a tiny eye or set a sleeve smoothly into the armhole of a child's garment, you can appreciate how small hearts and tiny arteries intensify the technical challenge and potential risk of invasive management for women. In such cases, drug therapy is an attractive, low-risk option.

Just twenty years ago, drugs could do little more than control heart disease symptoms and, at best, keep patients free of pain. But in recent years, drug options have mushroomed. With new classifications of drugs and a growing range of choices within each classification, medication can now treat the underlying problem and protect the heart. True, cardiac medications, like all other medications, have side effects, and sometimes these are intolerable. But because so many options exist, careful monitoring permits most people to enjoy the maximum benefit of drugs with minimal discomfort.

Nitrates

Nitroglycerin, the old standby and one of the only weapons in the cardiologist's arsenal until the 1960s, continues to play a vital role in the treatment of heart disease. In a scenario that has been played and replayed for generations, patients slip a tiny white tablet under their tongue at the first hint of pain or in anticipation of an activity likely to bring it on. Today, nitrates can also be taken as mouth sprays or time-release tablets, through the skin on patches, or, if you need intensive care, directly into the vein via intravenous drip. Regardless of how the drug is administered, it opens the coronary arteries, increases blood flow, and thereby helps to protect the heart muscle and relieve pain. Side effects—short-lived headaches, dizziness, and drop in blood pressure—are generally minor and most people tolerate them easily.

Calcium Channel Blockers

Like the nitrates, *calcium channel blockers* treat angina by relaxing the blood vessels. In addition, these drugs, which include nifedipine (Procardia), diltiazem (Cardizem), and verapamil hydrochloride (Isoptin), lower blood pressure and diminish the force of the heart's contraction. Diltiazem and verapamil also slow the heart rate. Thus, calcium channel blockers ease the work of the heart in several ways and reduce its need for oxygen. Since calcium channel blockers lower blood pressure, they are sometimes prescribed specifically for this purpose. Because they also prevent arterial spasm, they are prescribed to treat variant, or Prinzmetal's, angina. They also slow certain rapid heart rhythms. (Prinzmetal's angina and irregular heart rhythms are discussed further in Chapter 7.) Side effects from calcium channel blockers can include headaches, dizziness, and constipation. But most patients tolerate these drugs well.

Beta Blockers

Beta blockers, the most common of which are propranolol (Inderal), metoprolol tartrate (Lopressor), and nadolol (Corgard), lessen the heart's need for oxygen. These drugs also lower blood pressure, slow the heart rate, and reduce the force of the heart's contraction, much as calcium channel blockers do. But beta blockers work differently from calcium channel blockers. Consequently, the two types of drugs are not interchangeable.

Beta blockers can be troublesome, especially for women. Although they are beneficial to most patients after a heart attack and useful in the treatment of mitral valve prolapse, these drugs do not control angina or high blood pressure in black people as well as they do in white people. If you are trying to lose weight, beta blockers can frustrate your effort because they slow the metabolism and keep you from burning calories. They might even make you gain weight. In addition, beta blockers can make you feel sluggish and depressed, lose your interest in sex, and keep you from sleeping. These drugs can also raise cholesterol, aggravate variant angina and asthma, and endanger people with insulin-dependent diabetes because they can mask insulin reactions.

Antiarrhythmics

Aside from medications that relieve angina, numerous drugs can effectively control other conditions associated with coronary heart disease. A number of preparations, including procainamide hydrochloride (Procan), quinidine gluconate (Quinaglute), and disopyramide phosphate (Norpace), which comprise a classification of drugs called *antiarrhythmics*, alter the patterns of electrical conductivity in the heart and thereby regulate its beat. Side effects from these drugs include dizziness, stomach upset, fatigue, blurred vision, difficulty sleeping, tremor, and rash.

Digitalis

Digoxin (Lanoxin), a form of the drug digitalis, is not classified as an antiarrhythmic, but is sometimes used to treat arrhythmias, particularly when the heart tends to beat too quickly. Digitalis, which is derived from the foxglove plant and has been used to treat heart conditions for more than two hundred years, slows the heart rate by decreasing electrical conduction. Because digitalis strengthens the heart's pumping force, it is also used to treat congestive heart failure. However, the drug can cause the heart to skip or slow too much. Other side effects include nausea, loss of appetite, and visual disturbances.

ACE Inhibitors

Drugs such as ramipril (Altace), captopril (Capoten), lisinopril (Prinivil), and enalapril maleate (Vasotec) provide other options for treating heart failure and high blood pressure. (Heart failure is discussed further in Chapter 7.) These formulations prevent certain enzyme changes that constrict the blood vessels and encourage fluid and sodium retention. By keeping the vessels open and reducing fluid volume in the blood, these drugs indirectly support the sluggish muscle and improve its ability to dispatch blood. ACE inhibitors can harm developing babies and therefore should not be taken by pregnant women. ACE inhibitors are also less effective in black people. They can cause a range of side effects, most of them minor, including cough, skin rash, loss of taste and appetite, weakness, fluid retention, palpitations, and headaches.

Other Drug Options

Several other types of drugs are often prescribed to augment treatment. *Anticoagulants* (such as warfarin [Coumadin] are useful in preventing blood clots; *diuretics* (such as chlorothiazide [Diuril] or furosemide [Lasix]) aid in flushing excess fluid from the body; and *hemorrheologic agents* (such as pentoxifylline [Trental]) improve circulation. All in all, drugs provide abundant and varied options for controlling the heartbeat, improving the heart's pumping ability, and facilitating circulation within the heart and throughout the body. As a result, drug therapy has protected the health and enhanced the lifestyle of millions of women with heart disease.

What You Should Know About Your Medications

This is not to say that finding the best drug in the best dose for any one patient is an easy or instant task. Older people are more sensitive to drugs than younger people; smaller people need smaller dosages than larger people; and recommended dosages are based largely on trials in middle-aged men, who are larger and younger than most of the women for whom these medications are prescribed. Consequently, identifying the best prescription for you may take some trial and error.

You can speed the process by assuming an active partnership with your doctor. When your physician prescribes a new medication, make sure you understand the drug well enough to evaluate how it is affecting you. What is this medication supposed to do? How can you tell if it is working? What physical and psychological side effects can you expect? (Constipation? Drowsiness? Stomach upset? Depression? Loss of sexual desire?) What plan does your physician have to adjust or change your medication to achieve the optimum benefit with the minimum adverse reaction?

In addition, whenever you get a new medication, be sure you know exactly how to take it. Should you take the drug with food? On an empty stomach? What should you do if you miss a dose? What if you can't remember when you last took the drug? Find out if there is any food, beverage, or other drug you should be sure to take with this drug. If you are taking diuretics, for example, you may need to make a concerted effort to eat foods high in potassium (such as bananas, oranges, and tomatoes) to compensate for the potassium the diuretics tend to flush from your body. Conversely, ask whether any of your medications is incompatible with any food, beverage (including alcohol), or other medication.

Drugs can cost a fortune, and in an attempt to contain expense, you may be able to take a generic preparation rather than a name brand. But don't automatically assume that you can. Sometimes, the chemical composition of the generic is just dissimilar enough to make a difference. Other times, the binding agents that hold the name brand, but not the generic, tablet together are critical to the way your body utilizes the drug. Whether a generic is acceptable varies not only from drug to drug but also from condition to condition for which the drug is prescribed. If you are interested in using a generic preparation—even aspirin—check with your physician first.

When you begin taking any new drug, pay attention to how you feel. Beyond being alert to whether the drug is working, are you different in any way? Are you sleeping more or less? Are you confused? Lethargic? Unusually hungry? Are you sneezing? Coughing? Going to the bathroom more frequently? Jot down your observations even if they seem unrelated and go over them the next time you see your physician. Drugs sometimes work in strange ways, and the more

SOME COMMON CARDIAC DRUGS*

DRUG (COMMON BRAND NAMES)	WHAT THEY DO	WHEN USED
Nitrates		
Cardilate	dilate coronary arteries;	to treat angina;
Ismo	increase blood flow out	congestive heart failure
Iso-Bid	of heart	
Nitro-Bid		
Nitrostat		
Transderm-Nitro		
Nitro-Dur		
Calcium Channel Blockers		
Procardia	dilate coronary arteries;	to treat angina and
Cardizem	slow heart rate; reduce	variant angina; some
Calan	force of contraction;	arrhythmias; high blood
Isoptin	control spasm	pressure; migraine
Cardene		headache
Verelan		
Plendil		
Beta Blockers		
Inderal	lower blood pressure;	to treat angina; high
Lopressor	slow heart rate;	blood pressure; some
Corgard	reduce force of	arrhythmias; mitral valve
Sectral	contraction; help	prolapse; migraine
	prevent recurrent heart	headache
	attack	

Antiarrhythmics

Procan	regulate heart rhythm	to correct irregular heart
Quinaglute		rhythm
Quinidex		
Norpace		
Tambocor		
Tonocard		
Ethmozine		
Rythmol		
Mexitil		

Digitalis

| Lanoxin | control abnormal heartbeat; increase strength of heart's contraction | to treat rapid or irregular heart rhythm; congestive heart failure |

ACE Inhibitors

Altace	prevent constriction of blood vessels; prevent retention of sodium and fluid	to treat congestive heart failure; high blood pressure
Capoten		
Lotensin		
Prinivil		
Vasotec		
Zestril		

Diuretics

Aldactone	increase excretion of sodium and fluid	to treat congestive heart failure; high blood pressure
Bumex		
Diuril		
Dyazide		
Dyrenium		
HydroDIURIL		
Lasix		
Zaroxolyn		
Maxzide		

Anticoagulants

| Coumadin | slow clotting action of blood | to prevent clots caused by heart attacks, atrial fibrillation, some artificial heart valves |

Platelet
Inhibitors

aspirin	reduce stickiness of	to prevent heart attack,
Persantine	blood platelets	stroke; discourage
		clotting after heart and
		blood vessel surgery

---

* For more complete information, including side effects, see the Appendix.

precisely you can describe how your drugs are affecting you, the more meticulously your physician can regulate your dosage.

Generally speaking, it takes three days before a drug's effectiveness can be judged reliably. Thereafter, adjustments in dosage or preparation can be made every three days to three weeks if your symptoms resist control. Although adjusting medications may require patience and persistence, the process is ultimately successful for most patients. Therefore, unless and until a lesion obstructs most of a coronary artery, drug therapy is the option to choose.

Disease rarely presents itself in distinct best-case and worst-case scenarios. But for the sake of clarity, let's look at a patient whose condition sharply contrasts Bernice's.

BYPASS SURGERY

Eighty-two-year-old Harriet Silber, who was introduced in Chapter 3, came to AHI complaining of chronic angina. Her catheterization showed a three-inch stretch of plaque blocking the artery that serves the right side of her heart, a 75 percent blockage of one of the major vessels feeding her left ventricle, and a nearly total blockage of the circumflex artery, which nourishes the back of the heart. Harriet was a heart attack waiting to happen. Her blockages were too severe to be helped adequately by medication. The best way to protect her was bypass surgery.

When bypass surgery was first developed in the late sixties, the prospect of surgically improving blood flow to the heart conjured up images of mad scientists and furtive experiments. But within fifteen years the procedure evolved from a rash and radical undertaking to an everyday practice. By conservative estimate, well over a quarter million of these operations are performed every year in the United States alone, and for good reason. For appropriately selected patients, the surgery promises more years of active, high-quality living than any other treatment.

The Bypass Experience

The operation involves opening the chest and temporarily directing the blood through a heart-lung machine, which takes care of circulation while the heart is cooled, stopped, and repaired. Blockages in the coronary arteries are bypassed by harvesting an expendable vessel from elsewhere in the body (sometimes one of the internal mammary arteries from inside the chest wall, sometimes a large, superficial vein in the leg, and sometimes both) and sewing it onto the coronary artery so as to reroute the blood flow around the blockage. Once the repair is complete, the heart is warmed and restarted, and the chest is closed.

No matter how routine the procedure sounds, it is still a major medical event. Despite superb success rates for patients otherwise at low risk, nearly everyone approaches the event timorously. Many women are openly fearful. (Although men are just as frightened, they are more inclined to couch their apprehension in denial.) Whether patients admit their concerns before the operation or not, it is not uncommon for them to become uncharacteristically nostalgic, review their wills, or write soul-baring messages to their loved ones. One way or another they divulge that they are contemplating their mortality.

Fortunately, most professionals who care for bypass patients are sensitive to the patients' concerns and go out of their way to make the immediate pre- and postoperative experience as easy as possible. Before surgery, most hospitals have orientation and education programs designed to put patients at ease. The day before surgery, the cardiologist, surgeon, and anesthesiologist visit each patient; describe what will happen immediately before, during, and after surgery; and answer whatever questions patients have. In addition, the various therapists visit to explain their respective roles in the recovery process and to teach techniques for minimizing postoperative pain. This busy routine combines with the mind's natural defense mechanisms to ease feelings of apprehension effectively. With the addition of preoperative sedation, most patients go into the operating room feeling confident and calm.

As soon as the operation is over, patients are taken to the intensive care unit, where vigilant professionals and state-of-the-art technology protect them from impending complication. The expert care available in modern ICUs deserves much of the credit for the extraordinary success rate of bypass surgery. Yet this immediate postoperative period can be quite uncomfortable. Patients commonly regain consciousness while they are still hooked up to the respirator that supports their breathing during the early postoperative hours. Between the breathing tube, painful incisions, and general discomfort, this is not a happy time.

Not long ago, this discomfort was exacerbated by the very setup of the ICU. Almost always these were windowless wards that were brightly lit, noisy around the clock, and conducive to anything but rest. Happily, modernization is curing many ICU ills. In many hospitals, the traditional open wards are being converted into small rooms designed to afford patients the quiet and privacy they crave without compromising the attention they need. In the process, some of the most objectionable aspects of the ICU have been eliminated: the inability to distinguish night from day and the disorientation that often accompanies it, the disturbing cacophony of ICU routine, and the indignity of being bedded and cared for in a public place.

Aside from the obvious—that intensive care eases patients over the most formidable postoperative hurdles—perhaps the best thing to be said about the ICU is that patients are out of there quickly; recovery is amazingly fast. Although patients can suffer setbacks and complications at any point during recovery, only a minority do. As a rule, patients are up and out of bed within twenty-four hours and out of ICU within two days. By the end of four or five days, most are strolling down the hospital corridors. Most patients are ready to go home just a week after surgery. In another week, they can go out for walks and gradually increase their activities over the next month or so. By the end of six weeks, most are well enough to go back to work and resume most other activities.

Although most people recover rapidly from bypass surgery, the recovery itself is characteristically arduous, with each phase of the process marked by specific challenges. Most patients say that the hardest part of early recovery is managing the respirator and that once they get past that experience, they feel they can conquer anything. Patients' second most common complaint is the pain associated with coughing. Because anesthesia causes congestion in the lungs, patients must make themselves cough and do other respiratory exercises to prevent pneumonia. But coughing and doing these deep breathing exercises make the chest feel as though the incision will split open. This cannot happen. However, in spite of pain medication, techniques to minimize discomfort, and constant reassurance from the nurses and respiratory therapists, coughing, walking, and other exercises can be very taxing for many people and require considerable effort for several days. Interestingly, patients who have also experienced abdominal surgery say a chest incision is not as painful. Many women, especially those who are heavy breasted, note that a good supportive bra eases the strain on the incision. In any case, by the end of the first week, pain diminishes noticeably. Moving and coughing become easier. Strength gradually increases.

Still, progress can have its setbacks. For weeks, sometimes months, strength and vigor give way without warning to overwhelming and unbearable fatigue. Patients complain that they cannot sleep, that they have lost their taste for food, that they have lost their memory, and that they cannot read, think clearly, or concentrate. In addition, this surgery almost always takes an emotional toll. Beginning about the fourth postoperative day, patients typically find themselves feeling suddenly despondent or emotionally unhinged or angry. These feelings periodically disrupt their lives for weeks. Serious depression impedes recuperation for many.

Patients say that knowing what recuperation entails together with a strong support system enables them to endure. Gradually over the months, their depression disappears, their strength returns, and so do their mental faculties. But patients commonly acknowledge that full physical and emotional recovery takes a year. (Coping with these problems is discussed more fully in Chapter 8.)

What Bypass Accomplishes

With recovery this arduous, one would submit to surgery only if the benefit made the discomfort worthwhile. The question then becomes what constitutes benefit? If benefit meant cure, the decision would be easy. But atherosclerosis is a progressive condition, and bypass surgery is a temporary measure. Depending on the number and location of blockages, the procedure can be lifesaving, at least for a while. In most instances, however, its intention is to stave off heart attack and control pain. In any case, the results are estimated to last ten years. In some cases, results hold surprisingly longer. In other cases, symptoms recur distressingly sooner.

All the research, which is based predominantly on men, has clearly documented that bypass surgery can save your life if your left main coronary artery is significantly obstructed. This vessel forms the trunk of the multibranch arterial tree that feeds the left ventricle, which is the most important chamber of the heart because it is responsible for pumping blood throughout the body. If blood supply to this chamber is blocked, death is swift and certain, so surgery to correct left main artery disease is imperative. This condition occurs more commonly in men.

Statistically speaking, surgery will probably also prolong your life if you have 70 percent blockage in three coronary arteries and minor damage to your heart muscle if you fall into several other high-risk categories, defined in part by age and the extent of your heart disease. Paradoxically, if you fall into one of these high-risk categories, surgery also becomes a bit more of a gamble.

In most instances, surgery is prescribed not to lengthen life but to prevent a heart attack and the permanent disability that it can cause. Whether surgery is advisable depends largely on the location of the blockages. If a significant blockage threatens a large or essential area of heart muscle, then protecting it from heart attack is particularly important. If the blockage lies in a less critical area, heart attack is a less ominous possibility.

Surgery is also intended to reduce or eliminate angina, thereby permitting more active, enjoyable living. But pain is not necessarily an indication of serious disease. As silent heart disease attests, people can die from a heart attack without ever knowing they've had one. Conversely, as syndrome X illustrates, pain can emanate from microscopic vessels responsible for feeding a tiny area of heart muscle. So pain can be an independent issue. How severe is yours? To what extent does it impede your activities? How successfully is it managed by medication? The answers to these questions will help determine whether bypass surgery makes sense for you.

Candidates for Bypass Surgery

When surgery is intended to prevent a heart attack and relieve pain, it is usually recommended to patients with blockages exceeding 70 percent in at least two vessels. But this is a guideline, not a rigid rule.

Many factors influence the decision, and sometimes they are personal rather than medical. Under some circumstances, elective surgery is clearly inadvisable. Ann Kromer, for example, was not getting acceptable relief from medications and needed surgery to achieve any semblance of decent life-style. But seventy-five-year-old Ann was newly widowed. When we saw her in February 1991 and concluded that surgery was her best option, we also realized that she was still grieving deeply over her husband's death. She was intensely sad, cried spontaneously, and suffered from insomnia. Moreover, she spent only her winters in Phoenix, where AHI is located; her family and friends were in Boston. We were afraid that Ann's emotional state might compromise her recovery from surgery, and we recommended that she delay the operation until she got back home, where she had the support of family and friends, and until she felt more like herself.

Sometimes patients themselves feel that the circumstances of their lives prohibit elective surgery. Doris Smathers, for example, was reluctant to undergo surgery even though it was probably her best chance for pain-free life. At age seventy-three, she felt she was too old. In addition, she had a seventy-eight-year-old husband who had cancer, and she worried about the upheaval that surgery would impose on their lives. Since surgery was not necessary to save her life, she was willing to go on taking medicine and putting up with whatever limitations angina imposed.

Some women, however, find the ever-present threat of angina unacceptable. They also find the ongoing need to take medication an intolerable reminder that they are "sick," and they would prefer to be "fixed" with a bypass operation. Although patients who undergo surgery must adopt new lifelong habits to stall the progression of atherosclerosis (see Chapter 10) and must commonly take medication indefinitely as well, some women find bypass appealing because they perceive it as definitive. They opt for surgery even when medication might manage their pain and protect their hearts as effectively.

Bypass Surgery in Women

Superimposed on all the medical and personal considerations of bypass surgery are the disconcerting data showing that women don't come through the procedure as successfully or benefit from it as fully as men. They are at least twice as likely to die during or immediately after the procedure, although their long-range survival is comparable to men's. They are less likely to achieve complete relief of pain, and they experience generally poorer health and complain of a broader range of symptoms afterward than men. In statistical terms, these consequences make being a woman a more striking indicator of a poor surgical outcome than any other risk factor.

Now, what do these statistics mean? Although women face at least double the mortality rate of men, the overall survival rate for bypass surgery is exceedingly high. While statistics vary among studies and with the overall health of the patient, mortality averages about 2 percent for men and about 5 percent for women. In other words, an average 95 percent of women survive.

No one knows for sure why more women die after surgery than men. Some suggest that there is a mysterious, yet to be defined factor of female gender that puts women at added risk. This hypothesis rests on statistical manipulations that demonstrate that when you discount the impact of age and every other indicator of poor outcome, female gender stands alone.

However, a greater number of studies reveal that women do poorly because they are older and sicker by the time they have surgery. Since heart disease strikes women later in life than it does men, the fact that they are older is understandable. As people age—men as well as women—they tend to be burdened with other disabling conditions that can compromise their chances for survival. In fact, women are more likely than men to have high blood pressure, heart failure, or diabetes when they go into surgery, and each of these conditions has separately been linked to increased risk. This older-and-sicker theory is further supported by the observation that women enjoy better success from valve surgery, which is a more complicated procedure but which women usually undergo when they are younger and healthier. If this theory were proven, it would make a strong argument for getting women to surgery sooner rather than later.

Quality of life is a separate issue, and difficult to measure. Fewer women get complete relief from pain after bypass surgery than men. If the scope of a women's heart disease exceeds the reaches of surgery, she might still have angina after the operation, for which she would need to take medication. Moreover, if she were disabled by diabetes, heart failure, and high blood pressure before surgery, bypass surgery would probably not restore her to a state of youthful energy. At least one study, however, showed that better than half the women fared every bit as well as the men. And on an anecdotal basis, many women find surgery utterly liberating.

As for emotional status, another component of quality of life, some studies show that women experience a higher rate of depression than men. Separate studies suggest, however, that when women have good emotional support and effective strategies for coping with the problems of recovery, they do quite well. The rate at which patients return to work is another common indicator of quality of life, and fewer women return to work than men. But characteristically women who undergo surgery are older than men, so this indicator might not be valid. If women went into surgery when they were younger and less disabled, this trend might change.

Both mortality statistics and quality of life profiles might change sharply if women were routinely referred for surgery before age and other disabilities took their toll, but just the opposite is happening. Research that captured headlines during the summer of 1991 documented conclusively that women are intentionally being held back from surgery. When men and women have identical cardiac profiles, men are more than twice as likely as women to be referred for cardiac catheterization, which is always preliminary to other invasive intervention. Research published earlier suggests that as many as ten times more men than women with identical cardiac profiles get this aggressive treatment. Obviously, many physicians have no intention of treating their female patients aggressively.

Why this bias in treatment? Perhaps physicians have been deterred by several studies published in the late 1980s alleging that, in up to 78 percent of cases in some hospitals, bypass is prescribed needlessly. One of these studies, which evaluated the appropriateness of surgery among 386 cases in three hospitals (19 percent of patients were women) found that 56 percent of surgeries were clearly appropriate, 30 percent may have been appropriate, and 14 percent were inappropriate. Perhaps the most shocking finding to come out of this study was that 1 percent (six patients) underwent surgery even though they had no significant disease. Clearly, either ineptitude or fraud was at work, a reminder that physicians are human, and that there are bad ones as well as good ones.

Aside from this shocking finding and its corollary—that no one should undergo bypass without a clear understanding of the status of her own disease and the benefits and risk of surgery—the validity of these studies is questionable for several reasons. One, most of the research assessing the merits of surgery simply looked at who lived longer: patients who had bypass or patients with comparable disease who took medication. These studies found that in most instances patients treated with medication lived just as long. But surgery is usually intended to reduce a person's pain and improve his or her feelings of well-being, not to prolong life. Could the patients who took medication live as actively? Were they as free from angina? The studies did not address these questions. Two, for the most part, the research reviewed the treatment of low-risk men, and it would be fallacious to apply these findings to everyone. Three, in order to evaluate the long-term effects of bypass, the researchers had to review operations performed over a decade ago. But surgical technique has improved markedly in the last ten years. In particular, surgeons have come to rely increasingly on the internal mammary artery for fashioning bypass grafts, and these vessels hold up considerably longer than the saphenous vein from the leg, which was used in the cases studied. During recent years, medications have also improved. Furthermore, some patients initially treated with medication have since undergone surgery and vice versa. In any event, as treatments are improved and the needs of individual patients change, research based on work performed over a decade ago loses validity.

It is unlikely, therefore, that physicians have kept their female patients from surgery because of this research. What other reasons could motivate them? Perhaps they are trying to be prudent. Perhaps they are put off by mortality statistics. Perhaps they are discouraged by the evidence that women continue to have angina and fail to experience a marked increase in energy. Perhaps they are dissuaded by the paucity of research. In the few studies in which women have been included, they have been underrepresented, and most of the existing work has not been analyzed thoroughly enough by gender to answer all these questions. Without research to show the merits of surgery, physicians may feel compelled to follow a conservative course.

Whatever the reason, delaying tactics are responsible for perpetuating a vicious cycle for women with heart disease. As physicians steadfastly treat their female patients with medication alone, the only ones who ever get to the operating room are those who have deteriorated to the point where they must have surgery or die. Emergency surgery—in men and in women—always carries added risk. If, by this time, patients have also suffered other consequences of advancing age and are confronting heart failure, their frailty would further compromise their likelihood of a good outcome. If they die or fail to recover fully, they reinforce the physician's contention that women should not have bypass surgery. And so the belief that women do poorly becomes self-perpetuating and self-fulfilling.

In the meantime, there is mounting anecdotal evidence that when this cycle is broken, even small women with tiny arteries do quite well.

Donna Atkins was a victim of the vicious cycle. She first became alerted to her vulnerability to heart disease at the age of thirty-nine, when she discovered her cholesterol level was nearly 600. She put herself under the care of a cardiologist immediately, before she ever experienced symptoms of heart disease, and he monitored her closely. As the years went by, she began to develop angina, and he prescribed medication. Within a few more years, she was feeling short of breath whenever she climbed stairs, an early sign of heart failure. Her physician continued to monitor her and prescribe medication, but Donna's condition deteriorated. Eventually, she was coughing up blood with the slightest exertion. Donna was getting sicker, her heart failure had become more severe, and still her physician insisted that medication was the only recourse.

Finally, Donna insisted on getting additional advice and, at age fifty-three, wound up having bypass surgery. Despite her size—she is only four feet ten inches and has such tiny arteries that she required a pediatric catheter for her angiogram—and her advanced heart failure, she recovered without complication. At this writing, eight years after her surgery, Donna's medication has been reduced to just a preventive dose of aspirin. She is well enough to walk three miles a day and do low-impact aerobics.

Harriet Silber, eighty-two years old and no taller than Donna, underwent bypass surgery two years after she first experienced angina. She was out of intensive care in less than two days and discharged from the hospital after seven. Whereas recurrent angina had made her afraid to venture away from home before surgery, six weeks afterward she was walking ten minutes a day and enjoying being back in the shopping mall. Her angina had vanished, she felt strong and vigorous, and her family observed that she was more alert and lively than she had been in a long time.

Cases like these—and there are thousands of them—illustrate that with a skilled surgical team and superior postoperative care, women do exceedingly well. These cases also support the belief that, to some extent at least, women have historically done less well than men because they have gone into surgery in worse condition. Moreover, logic dictates that if they get into surgery before their conditions deteriorate, statistics on survival rates and complications will improve.

It is important for research to confirm this hunch. To date, the necessary studies have been outlined, but to the best of our knowledge they have yet to get under way. In the meantime, since surgery can save women from disabling heart attacks, we believe that women stand only to profit by having surgery at the optimal time: when their disease is advanced enough to warrant it but contained enough not to increase their risk.

Is Bypass Surgery Right for You?

If your physician recommends surgery, you will want to make sure that this is your best option given your unique medical, emotional, and personal circumstances. The answers to the following questions will help you gain this critical confidence:

Why is bypass surgery better than angioplasty? Since angioplasty accomplishes the same objective as bypass surgery but imposes minimal physical and emotional trauma (a complete discussion of angioplasty follows), why is bypass preferable?

How risky is bypass surgery for you? What factors in your particular case stand as potential obstacles? How will your overall health affect your risk? How do your body size and the size of your arteries alter the picture? How do the potential benefits offset the risks?

What does successful surgery mean for you? When your doctor says he or she has every reason to believe that surgery will be successful, ask what success means for you. Will surgery prolong your life? Save you from a heart attack? To what degree can you expect surgery to control your pain? What medications will you be likely to need indefinitely? How long can you expect the benefits of surgery to hold up? The answers to these questions vary widely from patient to patient. Since your physician knows your medical history and your cardiac catheterization results, he or she should be able to offer you some educated guesses. Without a crystal ball, however, no doctor can make any promises.

Finally, be sure you understand what to expect from surgery and recovery. The older and sicker you are before you go into surgery, the longer each stage of recovery is likely to take. Based on your personal medical profile, how long does your doctor anticipate it will be before you can resume your normal activities? Feel like yourself physically and emotionally? What potential complications can you encounter? How likely are they to occur? Take your physician's answers as educated guesses and be prepared for some surprises.

If you feel uncertain about your physician's recommendations, don't hesitate to get another opinion. If you don't already have a copy of your records, get one now. Be sure the films from your cardiac catheterization are included. That way, another expert can review your case without putting you through the diagnostic hoops again.

Second opinions are so important that some insurance companies require them before agreeing to pay for certain procedures, bypass surgery and angioplasty among them. Moreover, companies that generally pay only 80 percent often pay 100 percent for a second opinion to make sure that the threat of out-of-pocket cost does not stand in their client's way. And if the second physician disagrees with the first, some insurance companies pay for a third opinion. Generally speaking, insurance companies pay for second opinions when they require them. Requirements vary from company to company and policy to policy. To find out about your personal coverage, check with your carrier.

While there is no question that second opinions are valuable, they can also be confusing. If necessary, get a third opinion and a fourth. Ultimately, you will pick up the threads that tie one respected expert's opinion to another, and you will feel comfortable about making a decision. While this process can be onerous and expensive, it is worthwhile. It may save you from unnecessary surgery. At the very least, it will strengthen your trust in the merits of surgery, and research suggests that approaching surgery with a positive attitude will help you make a smooth recovery.

Once you decide to have surgery, your cardiologist will refer you to a surgeon she trusts who operates in a hospital she respects. If you are so inclined, you can research surgeons and invasive cardiologists in much the same way you did a clinical cardiologist (see Chapter 4). To optimize your chances for successful surgery, a task force of the American College of Cardiology and the American Heart Association recommends choosing a surgeon who performs at least one hundred heart operations a year, most of them bypass. The task force further recommends that you select a hospital that does at least two hundred heart surgeries a year and that has at least two heart surgeons on staff. If you want to investigate the hospital further, you may be able to obtain assistance by calling the Public Citizen Health Research Group in Washington, D.C. (202-833-3000), a consumer advocacy organization dedicated to helping consumers make knowledgeable decisions about their health, or the Health Standards and Quality Bureau of the Health Care Financing Administration, in Baltimore, Maryland (301-966-6841), which tracks hospital mortality statistics. Unfortunately, revealing information is difficult to come by mainly because the current statistical reporting on medical and surgical procedures in our country is woefully lacking.

ANGIOPLASTY

Balloon Angioplasty

In carefully chosen cases, *percutaneous transluminal angioplasty*, commonly known as balloon angioplasty or the balloon technique, can accomplish the objective of surgery without a knife (Figure 5-1). In this procedure, performed in conjunction with angiography, a tiny balloon is passed on a catheter into the coronary artery. When the balloon reaches the blockage, it is inflated, compressing the plaque against the artery wall and eliminating the bottleneck. The procedure is performed under local anesthesia and is completed in about an hour. Patients can leave the hospital within a couple of days and are often back to their usual activities within a week. Angioplasty accomplishes exactly the same objective as bypass surgery with a fraction of the physical, emotional, or financial cost.

In angioplasty, the physician is guided only by fluoroscopic images of the coronary arteries. Imagine feeding a wire into a thin, winding tube of cooked spaghetti without snagging it. Imagine further working only by feel, and perhaps you can appreciate the challenge. Not surprisingly, when the procedure was first developed in 1977, it was cautiously performed only on very-low-risk patients whose angiograms showed a single mass of plaque strategically positioned within easy reach of the balloon and soft enough to yield readily to its pressure. Success bred courage, however, and within a few years, experts were confidently performing angioplasty on patients who had had worsening angina, heart attacks, more than a single blockage in one or several arteries, or bypass grafts that had closed up. Today more than 250,000 balloon angioplasties are performed on coronary arteries every year.

BALLOON ANGIOPLASTY

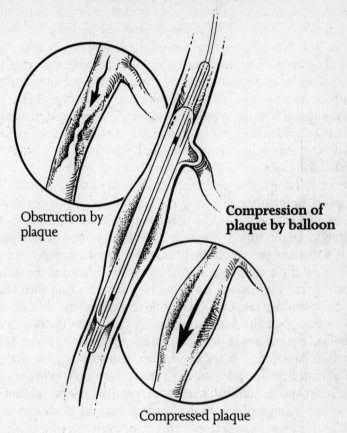

Obstruction by plaque

Compression of plaque by balloon

Compressed plaque

FIGURE 5-1.

Yet the procedure is no panacea. In some instances, plaque lies beyond the catheter's reach. Even if the plaque is accessible, it may be so hardened that the pressure of the balloon can't budge it. Or the bottleneck may be too narrow for the balloon to penetrate. Ten percent of cases fail immediately and may precipitate the need for emergency surgery, which always carries added risk. Of the remaining 90 percent, about 4 percent shut down within days and another third shut down in less than a year. When obstructions re-form, repeated attempts at angioplasty have sometimes succeeded. In other instances, bypass surgery has solved the problem.

Survival rates are impressive: 995 out of 1,000 cases. There is the remote risk that the procedure can induce a heart attack or stroke. For women, short-term statistics are not quite as good as for men, but women who successfully come through the period immediately following the procedure enjoy more long-lasting results than men. For good candidates, angioplasty is absolutely preferable to surgery.

Survival aside, angioplasty relieves chest pain better than medication alone, according to research published in January 1992. This study, significant because it is the first rigorous assessment of its kind, looked at 212 patients—predictably but not surprisingly, all were men —and found that angioplasty eliminated pain in 64 percent, while medicine alone worked well for only 46 percent.

Nanette Priester is the perfect illustration of what angioplasty can accomplish. She had been taking medication for angina for several years. As her angina got worse, her medication was increased, but ultimately even maximum dosages were inadequate. At this point, Nanette's cardiologist recommended triple bypass surgery, and she came to AHI for a second opinion. When we looked at the film of her cardiac catheterization, however, we saw just one formidable obstruction, and we felt it was amenable to angioplasty. Six days after the procedure, Nanette felt that her energy level was up 75 percent, and she was optimistic she would continue to improve (Figure 5-2).

For Ruth Pinna, introduced in Chapter 4, angioplasty was a ticket home after thirty-nine days in the cardiac care unit following her second heart attack. Ruth had been poorly managed. After a bumbled first attempt at angioplasty, Ruth's cardiologist was unable to wean her from an intravenous nitroglycerin drip; every time he tried, she experienced intolerable pain. Ruth seemed headed for nowhere, until she was moved to a different hospital and put in more competent hands. The second attempt at angioplasty worked. After the inflation of a balloon her pain was gone, and within three days her medical odyssey was over. In the intervening eight years, Ruth has had to increase her medication somewhat, but she continues to experience the benefit of that procedure nevertheless.

Auxiliary Endovascular Techniques

Because angioplasty is limited in what it can accomplish and bypass surgery is a major operation, researchers are ever exploring innovative ways to clean out the arteries and hold them open with a minimum of upheaval and risk. Today an array of miniaturized space-age

BYPASS SURGERY VS. BALLOON ANGIOPLASTY

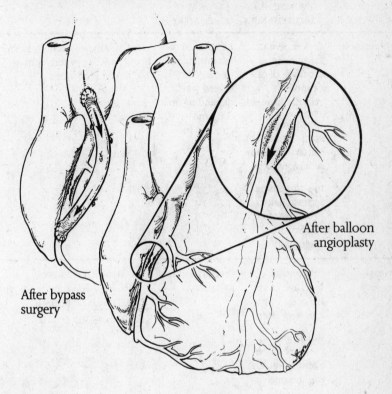

After balloon
angioplasty

After bypass
surgery

FIGURE 5-2.

tools developed for use inside the arteries is beginning to augment angioplasty.

This is the substance of science fiction. Just as Isaac Asimov's miniaturized scientists in *The Fantastic Voyage* traveled inside the human arteries, so the physician, using a camcorder no larger than a pinhead and watching the video it broadcasts on a nearby monitor, can "travel" into his or her patient's arteries and look around. Then, with a minuscule ultrasound wand, he or she can evaluate the architecture inside, choose the perfect tool, and develop the ideal strategy for repair.

When accumulated debris closes off an artery, lasers can open a

TREATMENT OPTIONS FOR CORONARY HEART DISEASE

TYPE OF TREATMENT	RECOMMENDED CIRCUMSTANCES	TIME NEEDED FOR FULL RECOVERY	COST*
medication	to compensate for minor blockage of one or more coronary arteries to relieve symptoms caused by minor blockages to compensate for residual problems after surgery or angioplasty	benefits can be felt immediately or may take several weeks, depending on drug and circumstance	varies widely with drug, whether brand name or generic is used, and how it is obtained
bypass surgery	substantial blockage of left main coronary artery substantial blockage of one or more vessels that are not amenable to angioplasty	several months to a year	$ 7,000 to 12,000 surgeon 1,900 to 2,300 anesthesiologist 25,000 to 34,000 hospital $33,900 to 48,300
balloon angioplasty	substantial soft blockage of one or more vessels within reach of catheter	several days to two weeks	$ 2,300 to 5,000 specialist 800 to 1,000 anesthesiologist 14,000 to 19,000 hospital $17,100 to 25,000
balloon angioplasty aided by one or several new endovascular tools	failed balloon angioplasty or complete or calcified blockage of one or more arteries within reach of catheter	several days to two weeks	$ 2,700 to 6,000 specialist 800 to 1,000 anesthesiologist 19,000 to 24,000 hospital $22,500 to 31,000

* Costs vary widely depending on geographic location, hospital, and individual case.
Source: L.B.A. Consulting, Inc., Denver, CO.

channel into which a balloon can then be inserted and inflated. When plaque, once soft and malleable, grows hard with age, shavers, razor-sharp propeller blades, and diamond-tipped drills spinning at sixty miles an hour can whittle it away and cart it off. When stubborn overhangs refuse to stay put against the artery wall, minute metal mesh scaffolds, called stents, can be deployed to hold them in place. All this inside an artery no wider than a pencil and as delicate as tissue paper! All this accomplished working by feel and guided by images broadcast from deep within the arteries themselves.

These tools have been on the drawing board since the early 1980s. As soon as researchers had seen the capability of angioplasty, they began to explore ways of removing the plaque rather than merely packing it back against the artery walls. The logical tool was the laser, a "magic wand" so powerful yet so precise it can peel the shell from a raw egg but leave the membrane and all its contents unharmed. However, what worked on eggs failed on human arteries. As heat from the early lasers vaporized plaque, it also injured the artery, and the concept was returned to the drawing board.

At AHI, we have been using lasers and other endovascular tools successfully since 1987. However, as the failed experiment of earlier years demonstrated, these tools remain in the embryonic stage of their development. In the spirit of the physician credo, "First, do no harm," we have taken on the challenge of these new technologies cautiously and conservatively. Since the coronary arteries are tortuous and the heart itself so indispensable, we use the new technologies for the heart only after we've used them successfully and confidently to curtail atherosclerosis in the large, straight arteries elsewhere in the body. It is in these arteries that we are doing some of the most dramatic endovascular work today.

When used in arteries of the heart, endovascular devices can salvage failed angioplasty, as they did for Wanda Ferris, the water skier who was introduced in Chapter 3.

Shortly after chest pain first set in, Wanda was treated with conventional angioplasty, and she thought she had experienced a miracle. The chest pain that had put a halt to her athletic activities was gone, and she was outperforming everyone else on the treadmill in cardiac rehabilitation. "I felt great and could do anything," Wanda recalled, and presumed her heart disease was a thing of the past. But in ten short weeks, the familiar pain was back, curtailing her activities and shaking her confidence.

She underwent a second angioplasty, which took care of her pain again. But angina is disconcerting, and patients' confidence can be fragile. As time passed and Wanda felt fine, however, she gradually stopped looking for pain lurking in the shadows. Ten weeks passed; no pain. Three months passed; no pain. But at the five-month mark, Wanda was stricken once again.

We believed a stent would hold her artery open, but we approached the idea with caution. The arteries of the heart bend and twist, but the only stent available at the time was relatively stiff. In addition, Wanda is a small woman, and her little arteries would heighten our challenge.

The effort was successful, though not without complications. To accomplish the procedure, we had to make a puncture opening into the femoral artery. Ordinarily, this wound begins to heal when prolonged pressure is applied after the procedure is over. In Wanda's case, however, the blood-thinning drugs she needed to keep clots from forming around the metal stent prevented the opening from healing. The problem resisted correction for weeks. In the end, it cleared up, but it serves as a reminder that, intriguing and exciting though these devices are, they are fraught with potential danger.

Unlike Wanda, another patient with failed angioplasty hoped to be helped with a stent, but the architecture of her coronary arteries was simply too tortuous to accommodate the stiff stent available then. We tried and tried to tease that stent into position only to fail in the end. As the patient was wheeled off to bypass surgery, we bemoaned the limitations of technology. The kind of stent we needed became available less than a year later. In another five years, the stents we are using now will be obsolete, and future developments will permit us to accomplish feats we can only dream about today. Similarly, we have abandoned the lasers we used four years ago for superior types. And we have discovered that lasers currently available do not work well for cleaning the plaque out of an artery. Rather, they work best to bore a narrow channel through the plaque when an artery has been completely blocked. Then, we go in with a cutting device to drill or shave away the bulk of plaque. As we learn more and technology improves, endovascular capabilities will likewise improve.

At present, lasers and other devices have been used in only about four thousand patients—about two thousand coronary artery cases and the remainder in peripheral arteries. While the technology is widely available for use in the peripheral arteries, its application to the coronary arteries is restricted to some sixteen centers that are participating in FDA-controlled clinical investigation.

Since these endovascular techniques are so new, it is impossible to know how they will hold up under the test of time. Case studies number in the hundreds at best, and results are measured in months, perhaps a year. Unfortunately, it looks as though women are more likely than men to encounter serious complications after atherectomy, just as women experience higher rates of complication after bypass and simple balloon angioplasty. These were the conclusions of a 1992 Cleveland Clinic study of 276 men and 81 women. While the pattern is troubling, success rates for women were still substantially better than 90 percent, and we feel encouraged by preliminary results. And although the new technologies require millions of dollars' worth of equipment, these procedures cost the patient less than a bypass.

If you are referred for angioplasty, make sure you understand what the procedure can accomplish in your case. Will it eliminate your pain? (The answer to this question depends, in part, on whether all your blockages can be tackled.) How likely is it that the procedure will succeed for the short term? For the long term? (The answers to these questions depend partly on the architecture of your arteries and the degree to which your blockages are calcified.) What is the likelihood that you will suffer a heart attack or die during the procedure? What other complications might you encounter? (Aside from statistical trends, the answers to these questions depend on the particular dynamics of your heart and overall health.)

The skill of the invasive cardiologist can make all the difference between success and failure of this delicate procedure. If you are referred for angioplasty, your cardiologist will probably recommend an invasive cardiologist to you, but you can double-check his or her references (see "Choosing a Cardiologist" in Chapter 4). If you can, find out if this specialist's track record is at least as good as the national average: approximately one death per 1,000 cases. If you are contemplating using one of the new technologies, make sure your specialist didn't just learn the technique at a continuing education seminar last week; ask how many of the operations he or she has performed. In addition, make sure that the hospital is equipped to do bypass surgery in case an emergency arises and that a well-respected heart surgeon is standing by.

CHANGING YOUR RISK FACTORS

Whether your heart disease is treated with angioplasty, bypass surgery, or medication, you will get the best results if you live a heart-healthy life. If you smoke, you must find a way to stop. Cigarettes are so incompatible with heart disease treatments that some heart surgeons refuse to perform bypass operations on smokers unless they vow to quit. Likewise, a high-fat diet, sedentary habits, and unchecked stress will speed the accumulation of plaque in your arteries, and no matter what kind of treatment your physician prescribes, your heart disease will gallop forward. But if you give up cigarettes, trim the fat from your diet, exercise moderately, and hold stress in check, you will starve the mechanism that feeds your disease. The payoff: less pain, more strength, greater vitality.

This theory is not new. Beginning in 1939, researchers at Duke University, then considered radical thinkers, gave new life to patients dying from heart disease by putting them on diets consisting almost exclusively of rice. Decades later, Nathan Pritikin and his ilk also discovered that when people with crippling heart disease began living healthfully, their symptoms disappeared. At AHI we experienced the same miracle with the patients who adopted the Diethrich Program, a life-style program discussed in Chapter 10.

When we began the Diethrich Program, angiographic studies had helped us deduce that healthy living encourages the heart to grow its own bypasses. This *collateral circulation* improves blood flow to areas of the heart that would otherwise be deprived. But beyond this deduction, there was little scientific evidence to support our practice. Then in 1990, research finally proved that you can actually turn heart disease around if you lower your risk factors enough. In one test of the combined effects of a low-fat diet and two cholesterol-lowering drugs (colestipol [Colestid] and niacin), treatment shrank atherosclerotic plaque in 18 percent of the 162 men studied. Another study showed comparable results with low-fat diet and lovastatin (Mevacor).

Separately, Dean Ornish, M.D., and his colleagues at the University of California demonstrated that, in one year of healthy living, you can begin to *reverse* atherosclerosis *without* cholesterol-lowering drugs or surgery. Participants in Dr. Ornish's experiment followed a diet practically free of fat and animal protein, spent at least three hours a week doing aerobic exercise, practiced techniques to lower stress, and did not smoke.

Perhaps the most interesting observation to emerge from Dr. Ornish's work is that the women in his study, though grossly underrepresented, benefited from healthy habits most. The one woman in the experimental group and the four women in the comparison group showed more substantial regression (meaning that new blockages began to disappear) than any of the men (fifteen in the experimental group and twenty-one in the comparison group) even though the women were consistently less strict in sticking to the program. Even the women in the comparison group, who had not been asked to make specific life-style changes but were free to do so if they chose, showed some shrinkage of plaque, which was documented by cardiac catheterizations before and after the study.

Dr. Ornish's study was tiny and must therefore be viewed as preliminary. However, he has launched follow-up studies whose preliminary results confirm his early finding. His findings are intriguing for two reasons. First, they suggest that men and women who adopt life-style changes alone can improve and sometimes even reverse their heart disease. Some of Dr. Ornish's patients were able to eliminate all medications entirely. Second, his studies suggest that women are uniquely capable of avoiding heart disease. This inference parallels other research demonstrating that when women and men are exposed to comparable risks—when they eat the same fatty diet, smoke the same number of cigarettes, and don't exercise, for example—women are less likely to develop heart disease than men.

All these findings point to the same conclusion: You stand to benefit tremendously from good, clean living. If you've had bypass surgery or angioplasty, it will help your smooth, clean vessels stay open. If you take medication, you may well get to the point where you can cut back or eliminate it completely. At the very least, you are bound to feel better. At best, you'll turn your disease around.

TAKE ACTION

As you attempt to understand and evaluate your physician's recommendations for treatment, the answers to the following questions will help:

If your physician recommends drug therapy, why is drug therapy preferable to invasive management? What can you expect the drugs to accomplish?

If invasive management is preferable, are you a candidate for angioplasty?

If bypass surgery is recommended, why are you a good candidate for bypass but not for angioplasty?

What kinds of results can you expect from invasive management and how long are they likely to last?

How can life-style changes affect your heart disease, and how can your physician support your efforts to change your risk factors? If in doubt, get another opinion.

Regardless of which treatment your physician recommends, lowering your risk profile will enhance its effectiveness. Please: Turn to Chapter 10 and get started today!

CHAPTER 6
Treating Heart Attacks

Ihara Saikaku, a seventeenth-century Japanese novelist, might as well have been alluding to heart disease when he wrote, "There is always something to upset the most careful of human calculations." Since heart disease in women tends to develop gradually, you would think that preventive tactics could hold a crisis at bay. But the best effort of patient and physician cannot always stem the tide of advancing age and other influential forces. Despite diligent commitment to prevention, heart attacks sometimes strike anyway. And while they kill more people than any other illness, good sense, good care, and a little luck have enabled many patients to recover and lead normal lives.

Unlike angina, which occurs when circulation to the heart is disturbed briefly, a heart attack takes place when blood flow to the heart fails. With a clot lodged in one of the coronary arteries—or, on rare occasion, with a prolonged spasm of a coronary artery—circulation to the heart shuts down, part of the muscle is deprived of oxygen, and catastrophic events can ensue. The pumping action can begin to fail. Blood pressure can fall, impeding blood flow to other vital organs, especially the brain. Simultaneously, blood can back up into the lungs, threatening to drown the patient in her own fluids. The electrical system of the heart can give way as well, and as the impulses weaken or grow erratic, remaining pumping capability diminishes. At worst, the heart flutters, falters, and stops.

HOW DO YOU KNOW IF YOU'RE HAVING A HEART ATTACK?

We've listed the warning signs in Chapter 2, but they bear repeating here.

Know the early signals of heart attack:
- uncomfortable pressure, fullness, squeezing, or pain in the chest, usually lasting longer than two minutes
- pain radiating to the shoulders, neck, jaw, arms, or back
- dizziness, fainting, sweating, nausea, shortness of breath, or weakness

None of these symptoms certifies that a heart attack is in progress, but the more symptoms you have, the more likely it is.

If you know you have heart disease, presume you are having a heart attack if:
- you think you have indigestion, but your pain does not respond to antacids
- you develop angina that does not respond to nitroglycerin

If you suspect you are having a heart attack:
- Stop whatever you're doing and sit down or lie down.
- Take up to three nitroglycerin tablets—one at a time at five-minute intervals or as prescribed by your doctor. If the pain does not go away, call 911 or your local emergency number immediately.
- If you do not have nitroglycerin and have had symptoms for two minutes or more, call 911 or your local emergency number immediately.
- If you can get to the hospital faster by car, have someone drive you. Do not drive yourself to the hospital!
- When you get to the hospital, do not permit emergency room personnel to keep you waiting.

- DO NOT MINIMIZE YOUR SYMPTOMS. DO NOT DELAY. Waiting more than fifteen minutes to see if the pain goes away can result in permanent damage to your heart. At worst, it can cost you your life.

If you are with someone who appears to be having a heart attack:
- Do not permit the person to persuade you that her problem is inconsequential.
- Call 911 or your local emergency number immediately. If you can get the person to the hospital more quickly by driving, do so without delay.
- While waiting for assistance, make the person comfortable, usually by having her lie down with her head slightly elevated.
- Check for medical alert tags around the person's wrist or neck and follow any pertinent emergency instructions. Call these tags to the attention of medical personnel when they arrive.
- If you have been properly trained and the need arises, begin CPR and keep it going until help arrives.

CPR

Four minutes after a cardiac arrest occurs, the brain begins to die. If the patient cannot be revived immediately, she will die no matter what kind of heroics are performed once she is taken to the hospital. This fact was underscored when a noteworthy 1991 study revealed that of 185 patients who were not revived adequately at the scene of their heart attacks, not one left the hospital alive. In short, taking these patients to the hospital was futile.

On the other hand, if someone trained to perform cardiopulmonary resuscitation (CPR) is present when a cardiac arrest occurs, the likelihood that the victim's life can be saved increases dramatically. In the thirty years since its development, this technique of mouth-to-mouth breathing combined with the rhythmic application of pressure to the chest has been credited with saving the lives of 40 percent of Americans on whom it is used.

In cities such as Seattle, Washington, where knowing how to perform CPR is a common skill, where ambulances are routinely equipped with defibrillators (devices that deliver an electric shock to restart the heart after a cardiac arrest), and where paramedics are trained to use them, survival after a cardiac arrest is well above average. However, although late-model defibrillators with computer-assisted technology can be safely used by paramedics after brief training, fewer than half the ambulances in the United States carry them.

These truths imply that, once you have had a heart attack, your family or, if you live alone, neighbors and close friends should be trained to perform CPR. CPR training takes just four hours, costs only about $25, and just might save your life. For more information, call your local chapter of the American Red Cross.

EMERGENCY CARE

When a heart attack strikes, minutes can make the difference between life and death or full recovery and permanent disability. If you can get to the hospital within four hours after the first hint of trouble, six hours at most, you stand the best chance to benefit from emergency treatment to dissolve the clot that caused the attack. Ideally this treatment can restore blood flow to the heart before any permanent damage takes place.

Although additional medications are emerging, two drugs for dissolving blood clots dominate the market and have recently become the focus of controversy: The older, streptokinase, which occasionally causes treatable allergic reactions, costs approximately $150 per dose. Its high-tech competitor, *tissue plasminogen activator*, or tPA, is genetically engineered from a human protein, causes no allergic reaction, and costs at least ten times more. Is tPA worth its price?

Preliminary research, based on thirty thousand men, suggests that tPA dissolves clots more quickly than streptokinase. Since time is critical during heart attacks, it seems logical that the best drug would be the one that restores blood flow most rapidly. However, existing research does not prove that tPA saves more lives than streptokinase does, if used with aspirin and heparin, another blood-thinning medication. Follow-up studies never resolved the questions.

Those who use streptokinase contend that the differences between the two drugs are too small to warrant the disparity in cost. This, in fact, is the consensus in Europe, where streptokinase is widely preferred. However, in the absence of proof that streptokinase is just as good, most American physicians feel compelled to choose tPA. They feel that, even if this drug is only slightly better, the stakes are high enough to make the cost worthwhile.

Gradually evidence is amassing in favor of streptokinase. A study published in *The Lancet* in March 1992 showed that streptokinase worked as well and caused significantly fewer strokes, a common complication of clot-dissolving drugs, than tPA. The study involved over 40,000 patients in more than 900 hospitals in twenty countries. These findings confirm those of an earlier Italian study of 20,000 patients.

At AHI, we have been using tPA for years and will withhold changing our protocol until the debate is conclusively resolved. We expect final confirmation sometime after 1992, with the results of Global Utilization of Streptokinase and tPA (GUSTO). This study, initiated in 1991, is intended to be a definitive assessment of 34,000 patients. Since some research suggests that patients do best when they receive both tPA and streptokinase, GUSTO will also evaluate combination therapy. AHI is one of the clinical centers for the GUSTO trial.

Unfortunately, although GUSTO designers claim this will be definitive research, the published protocol makes no mention of any intention to analyze the study results by gender. Apparently, the investigators will not learn whether women and men react differently to these drugs and, if so, what to make of the differences. Yet the need for this information clearly exists. Although one 1991 study suggests that clot busters are equally safe for women and men, most other studies have demonstrated that women suffer complications, specifically strokes and other bleeding problems, twice as often as men, and no one knows why. Perhaps the disparity reflects an idiosyncrasy of gender. Alternatively, women might be at risk because their doses, which are appropriate for men, may be too large. Without research, there is no way to know, and to date no clot-buster research on women has been done.

For women, the most important issue may be whether they are getting either drug. Research published in the *Journal of the American Medical Association* in July 1991 revealed that these preparations are not given to men or women aggressively enough and that women are less likely to receive them than men. According to a second and more recent study, which reviewed the treatment of five thousand men and women treated in nineteen hospitals since 1988, women are only half as likely as men to receive these drugs!

When women are given the drug, there is some question about whether they get it promptly enough to do any good. Dr. Estelle Ramey, professor emeritus at Georgetown University Medical School, observes that because of potential bleeding problems, many physicians resist using these drugs unless they are certain that a heart attack is taking place, and it sometimes takes two days before the event can be confirmed by EKG or blood tests. Observing how emergency room physicians equivocate with their male patients, Dr. Ramey worries that since women's symptoms can be even more obscure, women pay the price for this hesitancy more than men. Yet speed is essential. Studies show that clot dissolvers given within the first hour after a heart attack can lower death rates by 50 percent. Waiting an additional three hours, however, can cut that benefit by half.

At AHI, we administer tPA, heparin, and aspirin, which reduces the blood's tendency to adhere to crags and clots in the vessels, while the patient is still in the emergency room unless she has had a stroke or recent operation, or unless she has a history of bleeding or another medical condition that would make clot busters dangerous. Fearful that these drugs might trigger strokes in people over seventy, some physicians have been reluctant to give them to elderly patients. Research published in November 1991, however, confirmed that clot dissolvers do not provoke bleeding in elderly people and in fact can improve their chances of survival by 4 percent. Since beta blockers can also save lives after heart attacks, we give patients these drugs within the first few hours of admission, unless they are in heart failure or we have an equally good reason not to.

Elizabeth Murray, seventy-three years old, experienced just this kind of care when she developed alarming chest pain and came to our emergency room. Treatment does not always prevent heart muscle damage entirely, and although tPA was not 100 percent successful for Elizabeth, it did keep damage to her heart to a minimum. She developed no complications and recovered rapidly.

By getting to the hospital as quickly as she did, Elizabeth could have received more heroic measures to protect her heart had the need arisen. Sometimes, angina persists even after successful treatment with clot busters. At AHI, patients who encounter this problem go directly to the cardiac catheterization suite for angiography and possible balloon angioplasty. When the artery is particularly constricted and lies within reach of a balloon catheter, angioplasty can improve circulation. If necessary, additional clot-dissolving drugs can be administered through the catheter directly into the affected coronary artery as well.

Because the heart is unusually vulnerable shortly after a heart attack, using angioplasty as emergency treatment is controversial and, to date, unsubstantiated by research. In the absence of data, some practitioners contend that angioplasty at the time of a heart attack is always too risky. Others feel that, in selected cases, if can help more than it is likely to hurt. Certainly, if the obstruction lodges in the artery that feeds the primary portion of the left ventricle and that critical area of heart muscle can be protected from permanent damage, the potential benefit is enormous. In any case, to minimize risk, only the vessel involved in the heart attack would be treated at this time. If the angiogram revealed another artery that could also profit from angioplasty, the prudent physician would schedule a separate procedure after recovery. By the same token, because of potential risk, bypass surgery and high-tech endovascular procedures would be contemplated during this emergency period only under the most unusual circumstances.

Regardless of the initial treatment, the next stop is the coronary care unit (CCU), where constant monitoring and intensive nursing are designed to minimize further damage to the heart. In the CCU, sophisticated technology and care can boost a patient's falling blood pressure, reverse acute heart failure, and assist the faltering pump. With intensive treatment, survival after heart attack has risen 15 percent, from 70 percent to 85 percent, since the inception of CCUs about twenty-five years ago.

RECOVERY

Once the crisis has passed, patients are moved to an intermediate care unit, where monitoring continues and their rehabilitation begins. Decades ago, rehabilitation meant a month or more in bed; contemporary treatment gets patients up and walking within days. At this point in recovery, you may get no medication beyond aspirin and a beta blocker. If there are no complications, you can usually go home within a week.

At one time, heart attack patients routinely underwent cardiac catheterization before leaving the hospital, but research has shown that unless and until patients develop angina, this practice is unwarranted. A light exercise test is routine before discharge, however. Although exercise stress tests are limited as a diagnostic tool, they are quite useful for people with definite heart disease. By walking on the treadmill at a measured pace, patients can find out whether angina is likely to debilitate them at home. Six weeks later, after recovering fully, patients undergo more vigorous and extensive testing to assess their status and determine whether they would benefit from angioplasty or bypass surgery. These procedures can relieve angina and protect the heart after a major attack, just as they can before.

Patients at AHI are discharged from the hospital with information and guidance on how to adopt a low-fat diet, exercise moderately, stay away from cigarettes, and keep stress in check. Statistical forecasts published in the *Annals of Internal Medicine* in 1988 showed that, after a heart attack, men who tackle their risk factors diligently can reduce their likelihood of another heart attack by 50 percent. Dean Ornish's study, in which women had the best results from efforts to reduce their risks, and other research, which shows that men are more vulnerable to the effects of risk factors than women, imply that women can do even better. As you reduce your risks, your heart pain will often subside, strength and stamina increase, and the need for medication is minimized. (See Chapter 10 for more on prevention.)

Our heart attack patients are also discharged from the hospital with instructions to continue taking their beta blockers indefinitely. These drugs have been proven to be lifesaving. In a pooled analysis of twenty-five studies, researchers found that long-term treatment with beta blockers cut death rates by 22 percent and subsequent heart attacks by 27 percent. Our patients also take a low dose of aspirin every day in an attempt to ward off another crisis. Data from several reliable studies show that aspirin can protect women during and after a heart attack. It also guards against strokes. More research is necessary to define the optimal dose. In the meantime, the best available information suggests that, if you have been advised to take aspirin, your doctor will probably recommend you take one tablet of buffered aspirin (5 grains or 325 milligrams) every day, always after a meal to prevent stomach upset. Taking aspirin regularly is not without risk, however, so don't take it without consulting your physician first. Furthermore, if you take aspirin regularly, you should also be alert to any bleeding symptoms, such as bloody urine or black, tarry bowel movements, and report them to your doctor immediately.

In April 1992, a four-year study of over two thousand men and women showed that the ACE inhibitor captopril (Capoten) can vastly improve survival after a heart attack. The drug, which prevents the heart from enlarging after a heart attack, reduced the subsequent development of heart failure by 36 percent and additional heart attacks by 24 percent. What's more, the medication did not interfere with clot busters or with beta blockers. The drug, which could save 150,000 lives a year, will probably join beta blockers and aspirin as lifelong treatment after heart attack.

When our patients leave the hospital, most are encouraged to begin walking right away, gradually increasing their distance and speed so that after four or six weeks they can walk three miles in an hour. After a week or two, they can also begin to do light housework, such as dusting and washing dishes. If they do not develop pain or shortness of breath, they can gradually increase the vigor of their activities. They can tackle more demanding chores such as vacuuming, return to work, and resume sexual intercourse in about three weeks. This schedule varies somewhat with each patient's age and the severity of her heart attack.

EMOTIONAL FALLOUT

Elizabeth Murray recovered quickly and smoothly from her heart attack. But emotionally the experience was shattering. She admitted that, for the first time in her seventy-three years, she looked into the mirror and realized that one day she would be gone. More than distressing, this startling confrontation with her mortality made Elizabeth feel almost childlike. She became weepy, dependent, and easily frightened.

Although Elizabeth was encouraged to walk around her neighborhood soon after her discharge from the hospital, two weeks later she still had not found the courage to go out. "I know my feelings were irrational, but I felt safe in the house. Whenever I considered taking a walk, I envisioned myself having another attack, and there would be no telephone, and I couldn't call my doctor, and I thought I would die."

Elizabeth's feelings were a normal reaction to the life-threatening nature of a heart attack. One way or another, most heart attack patients share these feelings. Another patient, a native New Yorker long accustomed to crowds and congestion, found that her heart attack made her phobic when she got tied up in traffic, especially on bridges. "I couldn't stand places where I couldn't get out. I'd find myself nervous and sweating, and I couldn't breathe. I just thought I would have a heart attack and I'd die trapped in traffic."

A third patient admitted that trepidation accompanied each new challenge. She was frightened at the prospect of leaving the security of the CCU and moving into a regular hospital room. The fear recurred when she was disconnected from the heart monitors, when she was discharged from the hospital, when she went on her first outing, and when she first drove her car.

For yet another patient, even imaginary challenges were threatening. Shortly after her discharge from the hospital, her cardiologist referred her for biofeedback therapy in an effort to help her learn some relaxation techniques. During these sessions, she would be hooked up to various monitoring devices, which assessed her physiological responses to the exercises. One time the therapist instructed her to imagine herself in an exotic place, and within seconds her blood pressure and pulse went haywire.

"The therapist told me to imagine myself in a faraway place, and all I could think of was collapsing thousands of miles away from my doctor."

These emotional responses normally wane after a few months. As patients force themselves to pick up their lives in spite of their fears, they discover they can leave the house, exert themselves physically, even endure the rigor and insecurity of travel without ill effects. In addition, they see that their strength returns, and with it comes their confidence. (Coping with heart disease is discussed further in Chapter 8.)

CARDIAC REHABILITATION

There is no question, however, that the recovery period can be difficult. To help Elizabeth through it, we recommended that she participate in cardiac rehabilitation, a program of progressive exercise, ongoing counseling to help her lower her risk profile, and peer support.

As with many other women her age, exercise had never been an important part of Elizabeth's life. Even though she had made an effort to walk regularly when the weather was good, she could easily rationalize skipping a day. Now, with her confidence shaken by her heart attack, we knew she would never adopt exercise as a permanent priority in her life unless she could be convinced that it was safe. Exercising in the supportive atmosphere of cardiac rehabilitation would provide the security she needed. By having a set appointment three times a week for twelve weeks, Elizabeth would make exercise a fixture in her life, a part of her routine that we hoped she would feel motivated to sustain.

Of equal importance, being in the rehabilitation lab would give Elizabeth an opportunity to talk with others who had experienced the same pain, procedures, and fears. This kind of peer support has helped countless patients to overcome their anxiety and to recapture a sense of security and optimism.

Elizabeth credits cardiac rehabilitation with enabling her to recover. She cannot overestimate the reassurance she got from watching the heart monitor while she exercised, and she admits that, without this reassurance, her fear of catastrophe would have kept her sedentary.

She also credits the nutritional counseling that was part of her rehab program with enabling her to adopt a low-fat diet. Although she had met with the nutritionist before she left the hospital and took a handful of printed information with her, she had lots of little questions in the ensuing weeks. Having a forum for answering these and the opportunity to share ideas with other patients helped her set a positive attitude. And Elizabeth believes that the peer support speeded her emotional recovery. "I sat in the house afraid to take a walk and convinced I was losing my sanity. Then I got to rehab, and I discovered everyone else had the same kind of feelings."

Women stand to benefit from rehabilitation every bit as much as men. Studies show, however, that women are far less likely to complete their rehabilitation, possibly because—and you probably won't be surprised to read this now—most programs are based on research about middle-aged men and therefore designed to meet their needs. While middle-aged men commonly need to exercise early and get to work, some women, especially those with family obligations as well as older women who do not drive and must rely on others for transportation, complain that the schedule of the rehabilitation center does not accommodate their needs. Women who see themselves as unattractive or unathletic feel self-conscious exercising in the presence of men. Sometimes, they need different exercises. When rehabilitation programs are sensitive to these needs, women seem to attend more diligently, look forward to their sessions, and profit from the program.

OUTLOOK FOR THE FUTURE

With cardiac rehabilitation, ongoing good medical care, and continued attention to reducing her risk profile, Elizabeth recovered to the point where follow-up testing one year later showed she had compensated fully for whatever damage the attack had inflicted on her heart muscle. On an anecdotal basis, other women, even those whose hearts were more severely damaged, have done comparably well. One seventy-two-year-old woman, for example, had her first heart attack at age fifty-one. Several years later, she had a second heart attack, more serious than the first, followed by angioplasty. In the intervening years, she also had a mastectomy, surgery for cancer of the kidneys, and a series of minor mishaps. Yet at age seventy-two, she continues to live alone, drive her car, work three days a week, and lead a busy social life.

Another woman, now seventy-six, had a heart attack followed by bypass surgery at age sixty-five. Her bypass surgery was fraught with complications. Her health is compromised by osteoporosis, diabetes, and atherosclerosis in her legs. Yet her attitude is positive and her life interesting. She walks every day, even though her legs hurt. Travel is limited, but she manages to visit her daughter in California and her son in Texas. And once a year she makes a theater pilgrimage to New York. Although medical care will never enable her to feel young and vigorous, she feels blessed with good quality life.

However, international statistics indicate that all too many women don't share these women's good fortune. One study, representative of many, found that twice as many women as men died in the first six weeks after a heart attack (9 percent as opposed to 4 percent) and that the disparity held throughout the first year. Women were also more vulnerable to second attacks. However, the reason why women are more vulnerable is unclear. Some studies point a finger at high blood pressure and diabetes. Another discredits the diabetes theory, but fails to propose any clear-cut alternative. One would expect that women's disproportionate rate of silent heart disease and their failure to receive streptokinase or tPA somehow play a role. Apparently, the explanation is complex and obscure.

So the search for cause must continue. In the meantime, as our patients illustrate, the best defense is prompt and vigorous treatment.

TAKE ACTION

After you recover from a heart attack, you may find that you continue to have intermittent pain or shortness of breath. Your physician will probably be able to alleviate your symptoms at least partially by adjusting your medications. You can help by keeping careful track of your symptoms and reporting them fully and accurately, and by adapting the kinds of habits that help ward off pain and a second attack.

Even when treatment works, if your heart has been severely damaged, you may find some limits to how fully you'll recover. Ask your physician about the degree of recovery you can anticipate and how long it should take for you to begin to experience it. Then monitor your progress.

If you find you are getting worse or if you feel different in any way after you begin a new medication, call your doctor.

Whether you have ever had a heart attack or not, if you have coronary artery disease, you need a ready plan in case you develop acute symptoms suggestive of a heart attack:

- Ask your cardiologist if there is any reason why you wouldn't be a candidate for treatment with clot busters, and unless he or she has a good reason not to, make sure your doctor plans to use these drugs for you.
- Discuss these drugs with your family and close friends and make sure they can act as your advocate in the event you are stricken.
- Know what hospital your cardiologist prefers and which hospitals in your area have the best reputation for emergency cardiac care.
- Investigate ambulance services in your community and find out which ones carry defibrillators and other advanced life-support equipment. Post the phone number of the company you prefer on every telephone in your house. Keep a copy in your wallet, too.
- If you live alone, investigate signing up with a company like Medic Alert or Life Call, which provides instant communication from a pendant you wear around your neck. Get a medical alert bracelet or tag that indicates your health status and keep it with you.

- Take a CPR course, and encourage family members and friends to take one, too. Take a refresher course once every year or so after your initial training.
- Know the symptoms of a heart attack in progress, and make sure your family and friends are aware, too.

Planning ahead could save your life.

CHAPTER 7

Treating Mitral Valve Prolapse, Variant Angina, and Other Conditions

MITRAL VALVE PROLAPSE

Some 5 percent of adult Americans, two thirds of them women, have a structural abnormality of the heart called mitral valve prolapse (MVP). Although other heart conditions sometimes cause MVP, most cases are thought to be inherited, since the condition runs in families. It can be painful and it can be frightening. But it is rarely serious.

Mitral valve prolapse is the term given to the exaggerated flapping of the two-cusp valve that separates the chambers on the left side of the heart (Figure 7-1). Under normal circumstances, the valve opens and closes without protruding into the atrium above. With MVP, however, when the valve closes, one or both of the cusps billows into the upper chamber. This abnormal valve action may produce a click that can be heard through the stethoscope. MVP is complicated somewhat, but usually not significantly, if the cusps fail to close securely, permitting some blood to leak back into the chamber above. This back flow, called *regurgitation*, is heard as a whoosh or murmur through the stethoscope.

A woman with this condition is usually diagnosed by chance when

MITRAL VALVE PROLAPSE

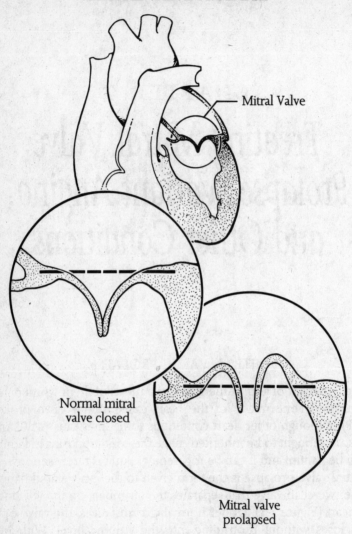

Mitral Valve

Normal mitral
valve closed

Mitral valve
prolapsed

FIGURE 7-1.

she is in her thirties or forties. While listening to the heart during a routine physical examination, the physician typically hears the telltale sounds and prescribes an echocardiogram to make sure. Echocardiography, the definitive test for MVP, not only confirms the diagnosis but also accurately assesses its level of severity by showing any structural change (usually thickening) and how much the valve is flapping and how well it is closing. Compared with other heart conditions, mitral valve prolapse is a usually straightforward diagnosis. Nevertheless, Dr. Richard Devereux, director of the Adult Echocardiography Laboratory at the New York Hospital–Cornell University Medical College, found that 40 percent of patients referred for one of his studies had been incorrectly diagnosed with the condition by their family physicians. This observation underscores the importance of obtaining expert medical care.

Patients with MVP are predominantly thin, particularly above the waist. Most have low blood pressure and a history of occasional palpitations. However, most patients with mitral valve prolapse never experience any symptoms at all.

When symptoms do occur, they usually assert themselves when women are in their forties. Under most circumstances, symptoms amount to little more than occasional palpitations, but for some people, MVP is quite debilitating. Some people faint, suffer chest pain, are short of breath, experience severe heart rhythm disturbances, and can be overcome with feelings of exhaustion and anxiety. In 98 percent of cases, even when symptoms are severe, the condition is harmless, and most physicians prefer not to prescribe medication unless symptoms interfere with daily life. Severe chest pain, shortness of breath, and palpitations can usually be managed by beta blockers, although these drugs can intensify feelings of exhaustion. When MVP results in severe arrhythmias, especially if it is accompanied by fainting, antiarrhythmic drugs can be helpful. (See Chapter 5 for more information on medications.)

While exercise has not been prescribed for MVP with the same consistency that it has for coronary heart disease, one team of investigators studied how moderate aerobic exercise would affect women who were experiencing MVP symptoms at least three times a week. For these women, exercise reduced the frequency of their symptoms and improved their emotional well-being. If you have MVP, exercise can probably help, and we recommend that you talk to your physician about the most appropriate program for you.

MVP becomes dangerous in fewer than 2 percent of women who have the condition. Curiously, MVP is more likely to cause trouble in men even though the condition occurs more frequently in women. If the back flow of blood becomes serious enough to cause severe difficulty breathing, the condition must be treated surgically. (For more on mitral valve surgery, see the section entitled "Other Valve Disease," which follows.) We cannot stress enough that this is rare. In another small percentage of cases, patients experience heart attacks and strokes. Again, such occurrences are rare.

For most patients with MVP, the greatest threat is an inflammation of the heart lining called endocarditis, which can develop when bacteria enter the bloodstream. The abnormal movement of the valve and blood flow across it can trap bacteria in the heart. To help avoid endocarditis, tell all your physicians and dentists that you have MVP so that they can prescribe antibiotics before any procedure that might cause even minor bleeding.

There appears to be no correlation between MVP and rheumatic heart disease, a complication of rheumatic fever that damages the mitral valve (see section on "Other Valve Disease," which follows), or coronary artery disease. By the time women are in their fifties, calcification of the valves, which normally occurs with age, commonly offsets the excessive billowing enough for the symptoms to disappear. While MVP is rarely serious, when it causes troublesome symptoms, MVP is not a trifling matter.

Samantha Mikinos, who has been aware of this problem since she was forty-two, first experienced symptoms after taking unusually demanding aerobics classes five days in a row. As she finished the fifth session, a sharp pain shot across her chest and her heart seemed to jump into her throat and begin to skip uncontrollably. Before long, the pain turned to a hot vise that grabbed her chest. In the six years since then, Samantha has discovered that the problem is most likely to be triggered by physical or emotional stress, and she tries to avoid both. Still, Samantha is periodically troubled by burning chest pain accompanied by depression and exhaustion. Sometimes, her limbs feel so heavy she can barely drag them around.

Although she sees some connection with physical and emotional stress, Samantha's MVP episodes are quite unpredictable. Sometimes they disappear in a couple of days, but other times they last for weeks on end. Sometimes episodes follow in quick succession, but she can go for months at a stretch without any problem. Sometimes her episodes abate gradually, and sometimes she just snaps out of them.

While an episode is in progress, Samantha feels wretched and has to force herself to remember that her condition is not dangerous. She becomes so sapped of energy that she must rest during the day and go to bed early at night, and she has to fight off feelings of depression.

But she finds that if she tones down her aerobics, she can go to work and keep up with all her other usual activities. Samantha turned down the beta blockers that her cardiologist said would control her pain and fatigue. "I'm bothered infrequently enough that I'd rather put up with the symptoms than with the side effects of the medication."

For Margaret O'Mally, however, who also developed symptoms when she was in her mid-forties, few side effects could be worse than the condition itself. The occasional fluttering that Margaret felt at first soon intensified into a thunderous thumping that was visible through her clothing. She never really had pain, but she could be racked with palpitations for days without letup. She would also awaken from a sound sleep feeling as though her heart had stopped beating, that she couldn't breathe and was about to pass out. Within seconds, these sensations would give way to incessant pounding, accompanied by such overwhelming anxiety that Margaret was besieged with cold sweats, stomach cramps, and diarrhea.

Margaret's anxiety came from fear, and it disappeared once her condition was diagnosed and she accepted her physician's assurance that she was not in danger. Although doctors once thought that the anxiety frequently associated with MVP was an abnormality of the nervous system, they now know that it is more likely to be a reflection of fear. Understanding quelled Margaret's panic; beta blockers regulated her heartbeat and kept her from feeling faint. Although Margaret still gets occasional flutterings, she leads a completely normal and active life.

Unless your case is unusual, you can work, exercise, even have a baby if you have MVP. During pregnancy blood volume always rises. Under some circumstances, this increase in blood volume makes symptoms subside. Under other circumstances, this increase could exacerbate symptoms and put a strain on your heart. To be safe, you should see a cardiologist regularly while you are pregnant. At other times, since MVP does, on rare occasion, become serious, you should probably have your heart checked by a cardiologist once a year. Otherwise, you can probably live normally in every respect.

OTHER VALVE DISEASE

As Chapter 2 details, valves are integral to the mechanical integrity of the heart. Under normal circumstances, they work as one-way doors to keep blood moving efficiently from the lungs, through the left side of the heart, out into the body, back through the right side of the heart, and then to the lungs, where the process begins again. If the valves fail to function well, either because they have become stiff and cannot open fully, or because they have begun to leak and fail to keep the blood moving forward, the heart's pumping capability is compromised.

Valve disorders usually affect the aortic valve, located at the exit of the left ventricle, and/or the mitral valve. Deterioration can occur from a number of causes. As patients age, calcium accumulates on the valves, stiffening them and keeping them from opening fully. Infections such as subacute bacterial endocarditis can also destroy valve tissue. This plus severe mitral valve prolapse and its accompanying regurgitation comprise the most common causes of serious valve disease in the United States. Worldwide, the most common cause of valve disease is rheumatic fever, the lingering complication of strep throat, or other infections caused by streptococcal bacteria. Although the mechanism by which the heart is affected during rheumatic fever is not fully understood, researchers suspect that, in an attempt to destroy the bacteria, the body becomes confused and attacks itself. This *autoimmune response* can continue long after the acute phase of the disease subsides and eventually takes its toll on the valves. While rheumatic fever has all but disappeared in industrialized nations, many adults over fifty had the disease when they were children, and they endure its legacy today.

As mitral valve prolapse illustrates, valve disease can be so slight as to be insignificant. In fact, the valves can function in a slightly stiffened or leaky state for years without causing symptoms or threatening health in any way. At the opposite extreme, one or more of the valves can be so damaged that the heart beats unproductively, which can be life threatening. At this point, the condition must be treated surgically.

When patients with valve disease begin developing symptoms, they usually complain of mild chest pain, dizziness, and/or shortness of breath that comes with exertion. Although the symptoms may closely resemble those of coronary heart disease, physical examination and laboratory tests can distinguish between them. The first clues come through the stethoscope, since each valve abnormality has distinctive sounds that help to define it. A resting EKG is also revealing, since each abnormality is represented by a unique pattern of peaks, valleys, waves, and notches. Of all the noninvasive tests, echocardiography provides the most precise and definitive information. It reveals the dimensions of the opening, the thickness of the valve leaflets, the degree to which they close, and the efficiency of blood flow through them. The ultrasound also shows the size of the heart chambers and the thickness of their walls, both of which change to compensate for inefficient valves. Cardiac catheterization can complete the picture by permitting a quantitative assessment of the heart's ability to pump blood, but catheterization is not usually performed unless surgery is being contemplated.

Since abnormal valves make patients prone to endocarditis, an inflammation of the heart lining, anyone with diagnosed valve disease or with a history of heart murmurs or rheumatic fever should take antibiotics before having her teeth cleaned or any other dental or medical procedure likely to cause even minor bleeding. Beyond this precaution, treatment depends on symptoms. When they are mild, they can be offset with medications also used to treat other cardiac conditions. Digitalis, calcium channel blockers, beta blockers, and vasodilators are usually prescribed, the choice depending on which valve is compromised and what symptoms the damage is causing (see Chapter 5). Under some circumstances, antiarrhythmics might be prescribed as well. As long as medication can compensate for the faulty valve without diminishing your quality of life and as long as the faulty valve does not damage your heart permanently, surgery is inadvisable.

As valve disease worsens, patients experience a range of symptoms suggestive of inadequate circulation. They commonly find that slight exertion leaves them breathless and exhausted. They can easily become dizzy and light-headed, indicating that insufficient blood is reaching the brain. If inadequate blood flows reaches the coronary arteries, patients can develop angina, even though their coronary arteries are clear. Most cardiologists agree that when these symptoms become severe, surgery is in order. This is particularly true in the presence of *aortic stenosis*, stiffening of the valve between the left ventricle and the aorta.

Thanks to echocardiography and cardiac catheterization, the deterioration of valves can be monitored to determine the optimal time to operate. You don't want to go into surgery prematurely because, although success rates for surgery run close to 100 percent, major surgery of any kind always carries some risk. But if you do need surgery and wait too long, the heart can sustain enough damage that it will never work correctly even if the valve is replaced.

If you find yourself facing surgery, several decisions will have to be made: repair the valve or replace it? Which kind of valve is the best choice for replacement? Choices will depend on your age, which valve (or valves) is affected, and the extent of damage. When the mitral valve is affected, it can sometimes be repaired rather than replaced. However, the repair can be tricky and should be tackled only by the most skilled surgeon and even then only under ideal circumstances. A good surgeon almost never makes the commitment to repair a valve until the operation is under way, when close inspection permits adequate evaluation.

In most cases, valve surgery means valve replacement. When patients are elderly, they usually receive "tissue" valves taken from pigs. These valves have been biologically neutralized so that they won't be rejected by the patient. Patients tolerate these replacements exceedingly well, but the valves do wear out, usually in about ten years. Mechanical valves, made from titanium, plastic, and a hard carbon compound called Pyrolite, are much more durable. But they have a tendency to cause blood clots, and patients who receive these devices must take anticoagulants for life. Thus mechanical valves can prove troublesome to patients with bleeding problems. If you need valve surgery, your physician will help you determine which of these options is best considering your heart, your age, and your overall medical profile. (The experience of valve surgery closely resembles that of bypass surgery. See Chapter 5.)

VARIANT ANGINA

Just as heart disease can exist silently, causing no pain, so the converse can also exist: angina in the absence of arterial blockage. This variant, or Prinzmetal's, angina occurs because the arteries go into spasm. The spasm periodically pinches the artery closed, stopping blood flow just as plaque does. Compared with ordinary angina, variant angina is much less ominous. It is also relatively rare, accounting for just 1 to 2 percent of silent heart problems in the United States. Interestingly, the condition, which afflicts women primarily, is more common in Japan, where it is responsible for 10 percent of all problems caused by insufficient blood supply to the heart.

In contrast to angina caused by atherosclerosis, which is generally brought on by exertion, variant angina is most likely to appear while you're at rest. But this rule has many exceptions. Sixty-year-old Ida Long was diagnosed with variant angina after she complained of tightness in the chest, which she associated with stress and with lying in bed at night. Betty Churchill, diagnosed with Prinzmetal's angina at age thirty-eight, felt chest and arm pain when she exerted herself or became intensely emotional. Sixty-year-old Mona Staggart, also bothered by variant angina, complained that after exercise—not during it—she experienced intense, enduring chest pain that did not yield to nitroglycerin.

Diagnosis of variant angina occasionally happens serendipitously. If a spasm happens to occur while the patient is having an EKG, the tracing will reveal a characteristic change, called an elevated S-T segment, for as long as the spasm continues. As the spasm subsides, the tracing will return to normal. In most instances, however, the only way to confirm the existence of variant angina is by catheterization. During the angiogram, the drug ergonovine is administered, and if the patient has Prinzmetal's angina ergonovine can bring a spasm on.

Most people with Prinzmetal's angina have more spasms than they are aware of. In a few people, episodes can last fifteen minutes or more, and if they are severe, can cause heart attack, serious arrhythmias, a disruption of the electrical impulse that makes the heart contract, and even death. To guard against these possibilities, people with Prinzmetal's angina should wear a Holter monitor for twenty-four hours so that the pattern of their spasms, which tend to occur during sleep, can be traced and medications prescribed accordingly (see Chapter 4).

Prolonged, severe spasms resulting in heart attacks are rare, however. In most people, Prinzmetal's angina is more frightening than it is serious and it can be satisfactorily treated with medication. Calcium channel blockers have been particularly effective in reducing the number and severity of spasms. Ordinarily, people experience relief within an hour after taking the medication orally and within minutes after IV treatment is begun. As with many medications, it takes three days before the medication's effectiveness can be judged reliably. After that time, modifications in dosage or preparation can be made every three days to three weeks if symptoms resist control, if silent spasms occur, or if side effects become difficult. Once your treatment is regulated, occasional persistent spasms usually respond promptly to nitrates. If you also have atherosclerosis, your condition is more serious and you may require angioplasty or bypass surgery (see Chapter 5).

Until medication regulates spasms satisfactorily, you may need weekly medical supervision. Once your condition is brought under control, however, checkups every six months should be sufficient.

SYNDROME X

To meet the demands of physical and emotional stress, every cell of the body needs additional oxygen, which is carried in the blood. One of the ways the body meets these demands is to dilate the arteries so that they can accommodate a larger volume of blood. In the case of syndrome X, also known as *microvascular angina*, some of the tiniest capillaries that feed the heart fail to dilate normally, depriving the heart muscle of oxygen when it needs it most. Syndrome X is a transient condition. For a while, it may affect certain capillaries. Then it may move to a different site. Sometimes, it disappears altogether.

Like variant angina, syndrome X afflicts predominantly women. Also like variant angina, it produces all the symptoms of coronary heart disease, but exists in the presence of clear coronary arteries. Severe syndrome X is more disabling than it is dangerous. Despite the classic heart pain it causes, syndrome X does not cause heart attack or death because it affects such a tiny portion of the heart muscle. Yet syndrome X is one of the most frustrating of all heart conditions.

Until recently, syndrome X defied diagnosis. Typically, preliminary tests would all point to coronary heart disease, but when the patient went through catheterization, her arteries would be clear and would not go into spasm when provoked. At this point, the cardiologist would conclude that her suspicious thallium scan results were caused by interference from breast tissue and would recommend tests for gallstones, hiatal hernia, ulcers, and all the other conditions whose symptoms mimic angina. And as the patient continued to suffer, one test after the next would turn out negative. Ultimately, as so often happens when physicians fail to make a diagnosis, the patient would be referred to a psychiatrist in the belief that her problem had to be psychosomatic.

Now, however, we have learned to short-circuit this frustrating routine. By measuring the oxygen content in a blood sample drawn during cardiac catheterization, doctors can verify that parts of the heart muscle are receiving insufficient oxygen. Thus, we can confirm the presence of syndrome X even though the capillaries affected are too tiny to be seen. It is now commonly known that women who have a suspicious thallium scan and a normal angiogram may well have syndrome X and should have blood samples drawn during catheterization to make sure.

Little is known about the condition or how many people have it. We do know that a substantial number of women have pain severe enough to force them to change their occupations. In one three-and-a-half-year study of 159 people with syndrome X only one person had a heart attack and none died. But more than half the people suffered chest pain at least once a month. Pain caused almost half to limit their activities and sent nearly one in five to the hospital.

Unfortunately, the condition does not respond to heart medications as angina does. Beta blockers are ineffective. Some people have benefited from calcium channel blockers and nitrates. Preliminary evidence suggests that a better treatment might be aminophylline, a drug commonly used for asthma.

For people who are suffering from syndrome X, the still-unanswered questions can be plenty frustrating. But at least a diagnosis can validate their sanity and thus provide some consolation.

ARRHYTHMIAS

When the heart beats normally, an electrical impulse emanates from the SA (sinoatrial) node located in the upper right chamber of the heart, and makes the upper chambers contract. The impulse then travels downward, passing through the AV (atrioventricular) node, a regulating station that delays the stimulus momentarily. Then, as it reaches the lower chambers, they contract. This synchronized sequence causes the blood to move in coordinated, efficient fashion from the upper chambers to the lower ones and from there out of the heart.

Under a variety of conditions the electrical system of the heart can become impaired. The system can be damaged by heart attacks or valve disease. As a result, erratic beating, or arrhythmia, occurs. Excessive hormones produced by the thyroid can also be responsible for arrhythmia, as happened to President Bush. Sometimes the problem occurs in conjunction with a congenital defect. And sometimes the rhythm goes awry without any apparent reason. Depending on the cause, the heart can beat too quickly (tachycardia) or quiver uncontrollably (fibrillation). It can beat too slowly (bradycardia), or unevenly. Alternatively, the conduction system can be interrupted. In this condition, called right or left bundle branch block (depending on which side of the heart is affected), impulses that emanate from the top of the heart are prevented from reaching the lower chambers in a timely or efficient manner. Women tend to experience benign arrhythmias most frequently around the time of their menstrual periods. The reason for this occurrence is unknown.

Because arrhythmias can originate from so many causes, diagnosis can be a real challenge, and a careful history is a critical first step. The pattern of the arrhythmia—under what circumstances and how often it occurs—provides important clues to its cause and its severity. While the physical exam and various blood tests also contribute to the diagnosis, the cardiologist's most valuable tool is the EKG in all its sophisticated variations. In addition to having a resting EKG, most people with suspected arrhythmias wear a Holter monitor to record their heartbeats while they go about their normal business. By comparing the tracing over twenty-four hours with a diary the person has kept, the cardiologist may be able to associate rhythm disturbances with certain activities.

If their arrhythmias tend to occur infrequently, people can be outfitted with portable intermittent EKGs, which permit monitoring lasting from a few days to many weeks. When the person feels palpitations, she can turn on the recorder, which is no larger than a radiopaging beeper, to capture an EKG during the rhythmic disturbance. These recordings can then be stored on paper or played back from the unit's memory over the telephone directly to the physician's office.

All EKGs with leads attached to the outside of the patient's body have one drawback: They cannot capture the electrical signals from certain areas of the heart. When getting this information is important, miniature leads can be guided through the blood vessels into the heart itself, in a procedure somewhat akin to cardiac catheterization called an *electrophysiology study*. This test produces meticulously accurate information, which enables the physician to prescribe and evaluate treatment with utmost precision.

Like most other heart conditions, arrhythmias range from imperceptible and inconsequential to life threatening.

Depending on the exact problem and its severity, a number of treatments can restore the heart to normal rate and rhythm. Under most circumstances, the first option is medication: beta blockers, calcium channel blockers, digitalis, and antiarrhythmics (see Chapter 5). The choice of drug depends on the type and cause of the arrhythmia as well as the person's overall medical profile.

Although the antiarrhythmics can be lifesaving for people who have fainted during an episode of arrhythmia or whose arrhythmias otherwise make them vulnerable to sudden death, recent results of a major study suggest that, when the arrhythmia is mild, side effects from certain of these drugs, namely moricizine hydrochloride (Ethmozine), encainide hydrochloride (Enkaid), and flecainide acetate (Tambocor), are more likely to cause fatal rhythm disturbances than the condition they were prescribed to treat. These findings suggest that physicians must prescribe these drugs with caution. If you take one of them, *do not stop* without consulting your physician. If you are concerned about using these drugs, ask your physician how the results of CAST II (Cardiac Arrhythmia Suppression Trial II) apply to your particular circumstances.

Medication can keep arrhythmias in check for years, and although people sometimes feel their hearts beating out of rhythm, these episodes do not interfere with their activities. Some people feel more symptoms when they consume caffeine, which is contained not just in coffee and tea but also in chocolate, some aspirin compounds, and other drugs (see section on caffeine and stimulants in Chapter 10), or when they use certain decongestants, mood elevators, and bronchodilators. Certainly, if these substances aggravate your arrhythmias, you should avoid them. Otherwise, if the frequency or severity of your symptoms increases, a change in medication may be enough to correct the problem; people commonly notice a significant change in just a couple of days. Serious arrhythmias, however, can erupt in periodic episodes that are life threatening. You may need to be hospitalized and treated with intravenous drugs or defibrillating paddles. The acute episode may last several days and can be so debilitating that full recovery takes several weeks.

When medication fails to correct the problem, you have other options. The oldest of these is the pacemaker (Figure 7-2). Developed in the late 1950s to sustain the beat of a sluggish heart, pacemakers have permitted normal living for some two million people who would otherwise be disabled.

Today's pacemakers respond to a variety of individual needs. People who experience occasional sluggish heart rates can be fitted with a backup system to support just the ventricles. Eighty-three-year-old Emma Smith had this kind of device at first. But after a while, she began to get headaches and feel dizzy even though her device was doing its job. Her symptoms meant that her upper chambers also needed support. When Emma received a dual-chamber pacemaker,

PACEMAKER WITH LEADS

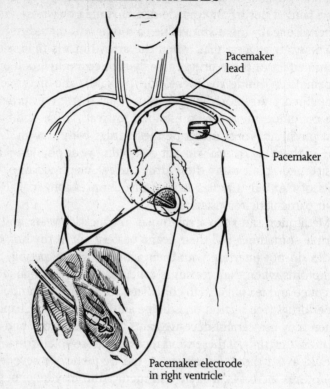

Pacemaker
lead

Pacemaker

Pacemaker electrode
in right ventricle

FIGURE 7-2.

which stimulated both the upper and lower chambers, her symptoms disappeared.

Advances in pacemaker technology have been extraordinary. By using a special transmitter and a telephone, patients can often have their equipment inspected without leaving home. Technicians reading the EKG can tell when a pacemaker malfunctions or the battery is wearing down, warn the person of impending trouble, and thereby prevent a potential crisis.

Technology is so advanced that pacemakers can sense a person's level of activity and alter the heart's rate of response accordingly. In a variation on this theme, pacemakers can respond to changes in respiration rate. Either way, they meet the body's changing need for oxygen and permit a wide range of activities. This kind of pacemaker brought new life to forty-two-year-old Amy Fine. Fifteen years after surgery to repair a hole in her heart, her pump lost electrical power. No matter what she did, her heart rate would not rise above eighty beats a minute. This woman, who was happiest trekking the Himalayas, suddenly didn't have enough stamina to drag herself through an hour's exercise class. Her pacemaker enabled her to work, shop, take care of her home, wander through art museums, and have energy left over for Jazzercise.

When the battery wears down, the unit must be changed in a minor surgical procedure. The life of a pacemaker depends on how much each patient's heart relies on it. Someone who needs only occasional pacing of the ventricles could go fifteen or twenty years without needing a battery change. In contrast, Amy Fine was told that, because of her consistent dependency and active life-style, she could expect her battery to last less than five years.

Just as pacemakers can regulate halting or sluggish heartbeats, so other devices can slow down racing hearts. Just as defibrillating paddles are used in the emergency room to shock the heart out of quivering chaos, miniature defibrillators implanted in the chest jolt the heart back into normal rhythm. Unlike pacemakers, which are implanted just beneath the skin during a brief, relatively minor surgical procedure requiring only local anesthesia, miniature defibrillators require open-chest surgery, with all its attendant risks and discomforts, so the miniature paddles can be placed directly on the heart. In addition, although the device has been approved since 1985 and over twenty thousand have been implanted in people worldwide, all the kinks have yet to be ironed out. The device sometimes fires inappropriately, delivering a painful blow. As the technology matures, problems are likely to be resolved. While its liabilities keep it from being used cavalierly, for patients suffering from ventricular tachycardia or ventricular fibrillation, rhythmic disturbances of the lower chambers that can result in sudden death, this device is lifesaving.

In fact, a landmark 1991 study of 650 patients who were on average sixty years old demonstrated that miniature defibrillators could prolong life for at least ten years. The investigators of this study estimate that, without the device, 30 percent of the 650 patients would have died within the first two years, about 60 percent within five, and virtually all by the end of ten. But in the ten years this study ran, only 40 percent died.

Because the track record of miniature defibrillators is so impressive, they are now being used in most major medical centers and, given the complication rate of some antiarrhythmia medication, may one day supplant medication as the primary treatment for these rhythm disturbances. Nine thousand of these devices were implanted in 1990, and the number is likely to increase tenfold or more if the results of other studies now in progress look as good. Researchers are trying to find ways to implant the device with endovascular techniques rather than in an open-chest operation.

In a newer approach to slowing the racing heart, electrophysiologists are blocking unwanted conductivity by cauterizing errant electrical pathways on the heart walls. This *catheter ablation therapy*, in which a thin wire is threaded through a vein to the heart, is successful in about 90 percent of appropriately selected cases.

HEART FAILURE

As medical advances enable more and more people to live with heart disease for many years, progressive loss of pumping strength has become an increasingly widespread problem, particularly among the elderly. Whether heart failure, which was first described in Chapter 2, results from a heart attack, chronic coronary artery disease, a separate heart condition, or prolonged high blood pressure, to one degree or another it alters the lives of some three million Americans. Women constitute a surprisingly large proportion of people with heart failure. In 1989, 642,000 Americans left the hospital after a bout of heart failure, and 339,000 of them were women.

Heart failure is the consequence of cumulative damage to the heart. At its mildest, the condition causes no symptoms and might be diagnosed only because a routine chest X ray revealed the silhouette of an abnormally large heart. The experienced clinician can often spot early heart failure by tapping the patient's back and listening to her heart and lungs. When the condition is at its worst, its telltale signs are apparent even to the casual observer. Affected people breathe rapidly. They look pale and sweaty. Their feet are swollen and their handshake is cold.

When the heart muscle begins to lose pumping power, the heart enlarges in an attempt to compensate. Like a rubber band, which rebounds with greater force the more tautly it is pulled, the heart tries to pump more vigorously from its stretched-out state. But the strategy doesn't work. As the lower chambers fail to move the blood along, pressure increases, and blood begins to back up into the chambers above. Pressure continues to mount. Blood on the left side of the heart backs up farther into the vessels that connect to the lungs. These veins become engorged, they begin to leak, and plasmalike fluid begins to fill the lungs. On the right side of the heart, mounting pressure is transmitted into the main veins of the body, and the entire venous system becomes burdened. Pressure backs up into the liver and the kidneys, which become weakened. All the while, fluid continues to build up, overload the veins, and leak into the body tissues, a phenomenon called *edema*.

In a second attempt to compensate, the heart begins to beat more quickly, but speed breeds inefficiency. Beating rapidly, the heart can neither fill nor empty completely. Now the heart is working harder and consequently needs more nourishment, but it gets less because the inefficient pump cannot keep the coronary arteries adequately supplied. And the downward spiral continues.

In the meantime, the kidneys try to offset their diminished blood supply by causing the body to retain salt and water, which increases the fluid volume in the circulatory system. In addition, the blood vessels constrict. These two adjustments effectively raise pressure in the vessels and move the fluids more efficiently. But the various accommodations further strain the heart and symptoms get worse.

Typically, people with heart failure become short of breath or tired from activities that never used to bother them. As they retain fluid, they can put on substantial weight. Once they lie down in bed at night, fluid may drift back to the lungs and settle there, making breathing difficult. If they've accumulated fluid in the abdomen or ankles, they may need to urinate frequently at night. When symptoms are at their worst, people can barely walk, and breathing even while they are upright becomes a chore.

Although unchecked heart failure can result in irreversible damage to the heart and ultimately prove fatal, astute diagnosis can lead to treatment that halts the progression of the disease. But diagnosis can be tricky. For this task echocardiography is the most valuable tool. Echocardiography can reveal whether the valves are at fault, permit observation of the muscle pumping, and identify areas of the muscle damaged by heart attacks. Echocardiography can also divulge the seriousness of the condition by showing which chambers are enlarged, the capability of the chambers to fill and contract, and the presence or absence of fluid around the heart. In addition, exercise testing is sometimes prescribed to measure how the status of the heart limits aerobic performance and to assess the effects of treatment.

When the pump can be fixed, heart failure can be cured. Andrea Winston, for example, developed heart failure when her mitral valve, which had been damaged by rheumatic fever, stopped functioning. As soon as her valve was replaced, the heart regained its capacity to pump efficiently, and Andrea's heart failure went away. Similarly, Amy Fine's heart failure disappeared when she received a pacemaker to compensate for her failed electrical system.

When the condition cannot be cured, treatment can often prevent the heart from deteriorating further and compensate for existing damage. Traditionally, digoxin (Lanoxin) has been prescribed to strengthen the heart's pumping force. Today, most physicians prefer ACE inhibitors, sometimes in conjunction with digoxin. While digoxin supports the heart directly, ACE inhibitors (captopril [Capoten], enalapril maleate [Vasotec], lisinopril [Prinivil]) work indirectly by keeping the kidneys from retaining fluid and lowering blood pressure. By relaxing the blood vessels and reducing the resistance against which the heart must pump, ACE inhibitors permit the heart to pump more efficiently.

A landmark study published in November 1991 demonstrated that the ACE inhibitor enalapril maleate (Vasotec), unassisted by digitalis or diuretics, can prevent the onset of symptoms even when the left ventricle has lost up to half its pumping power. This study, which included over four thousand patients and ran for five years, was the first to demonstrate that heart failure can be forestalled, and it will probably be responsible for a major change in treatment philosophy.

"Because of these findings, several hundred thousand patients with impaired heart function will be treated much sooner than doctors have treated them in the past," speculated David McCall, M.D., professor of medicine at the University of Texas and a member of the American Heart Association's scientific program committee. This study is particularly good news for women, since women are affected by heart failure more than men.

In another study published the preceding August, enalapril maleate (Vasotec) cut death rates in half (from 20 percent to 10 percent) for people with mild to moderate heart failure. The drug also helped to keep people out of the hospital. Other research has shown similar results for people with more advanced heart failure. The use of ACE inhibitors can prevent up to twenty thousand deaths and one hundred thousand hospitalizations each year, estimated Claude J. Lenfant, M.D., director of the National Heart, Lung, and Blood Institute at the National Institutes of Health. In addition, patients who take these drugs frequently find they have more energy, stamina, and a greater sense of well-being.

ACE inhibitors and/or digoxin together with a diuretic and reduction in salt consumption is appropriate treatment for approximately 70 percent of heart failure patients, whose problem emanates from the heart's inability to contract efficiently, a condition called systolic heart failure. For the remaining 30 percent, heart failure results from insufficient filling, a condition called diastolic heart failure. Patients with diastolic failure are usually treated with calcium channel blockers, which relax the heart muscle. Investigators are currently looking into the merits of beta blockers for this purpose as well. Sometimes people suffer from both conditions.

If you have modest heart failure, you may have to stop playing sports competitively and limit your heavy labor. But treatment is likely to eliminate your symptoms entirely. With medication to support your heart plus modification of your salt intake and a diuretic such as furosemide (Lasix) to rid your body of excess fluid, you will probably get over your shortness of breath and feelings of distention. If your heart failure is more advanced, you may need to cut back on your work schedule and rest during the day, and you will probably have to watch your salt intake more strictly. Sometimes, heart failure becomes acute and requires hospitalization. Treatment with intravenous drugs can often begin to turn the episode around in forty-eight hours, but if your condition is severe, it may take several weeks to feel like yourself again. If your condition is so severe that you are house- or bed-bound, you will probably find that, in addition to medication and a low-salt diet, using supplemental oxygen will ease your breathing and make you much more comfortable.

HEART TRANSPLANTS

In rare instances, irreversible heart failure, or what is often termed end-stage heart disease, can be managed only by heart transplantation. Today, this alternative offers people as old as sixty-five, possibly even seventy, unprecedented hope. Heart transplantation is clearly a last resort. Because of an inadequate supply of donor organs, many patients die before a match can be made. Rejection, too, is a problem, particularly for women. Yet 80 to 90 percent live one year after a transplant with good quality of life, and 60 to 80 percent live for five. Considering the alternative, these benefits are extraordinary. As medical technology becomes better equipped to manage rejection, heart transplants will become an even more viable option.

TAKE ACTION

Treatment for heart disease doesn't always produce instant results. You can help speed your progress by keeping a detailed log of your symptoms. What brings them on? What eases them? What do they feel like? How severe are they? The more fully and accurately you report your symptoms, the more your physician has to work with and the more likely you are to see results.

- Even when treatment works, if you have advanced heart disease, your progress might be limited. Ask your physician about the benefits you can anticipate and how long it should take before you begin to experience them. Then monitor your progress.
- If you find you are getting worse or if you feel different in any way after you begin a new medication, call your doctor.
- If you have valve disease, know which antibiotics you need to take before dental or medical procedures, and make sure that all your physicians and dentists know about your heart condition.
- No matter what kind of heart disease you have, be prepared for an emergency. Find out which hospitals in your area have twenty-four-hour cardiac care. Keep emergency phone numbers next to your phone and in your wallet. Know the location of the hospitals nearest to your home and office. Make sure your friends and family have this information.

CHAPTER 8

Coping with Heart Disease

Heart disease is not automatically cataclysmic. Thousands and thousands of patients have been swiftly diagnosed and effectively treated without physical disability or emotional trauma. But for every woman with a positive experience, there is one who has suffered medically and/or emotionally because of ineffective physicians, inaccurate diagnosis, or inadequate treatment. Even when medical care is impeccable, physical and emotional difficulties can crop up during a cardiac crisis, early in recovery, late in the game, or at any time during a chronic illness. Unresolved, these problems can persist for years. But with insight and effective coping strategies, you will find you can overcome seemingly insurmountable obstacles and that in the process, your anxiety will fade.

IT'S NOT "ALL IN YOUR HEAD"

For many women, problems begin before they ever get a diagnosis. Women complain that their physicians give them the runaround, fail to evaluate their symptoms seriously, and presume that their conditions are psychosomatic. The problem arises partly from the close alliance of chest pain and anxiety. In some instances, anxiety can cause chest pain, palpitations, and shortness of breath. The converse is true as well.

The problem is compounded by the truth that, although women go to the doctor more often and spend more money on health care than men, women tend to seek attention for minor problems while men usually wait until catastrophe strikes. According to one representative analysis, men went to physicians more than women for only one reason: trauma. For *all* other reasons—and they ranged from life threatening to medically insignificant—women were more likely to see their doctors. Researchers explain this disparity with a number of theories: that women are more interested in health; that menstruation, pregnancy, and other hormonal shifts make women especially alert to changes in their bodies; that because women have borne and raised children, obtaining health care is a way of life; that Western culture allows women to admit illness, assume a dependent posture, and seek help while the same culture trains men to be stoic; and that women's traditional roles leave them enough unstructured time that they can take care of themselves.

While the reasons are not entirely clear, researchers agree that the pattern exists, and it apparently has social and psychological origins. Substantial research also suggests that women suffer higher rates of psychological distress. For example, one fifteen-year survey of mental illness concluded that women have more "transient situational personality disorders" and psychosomatic afflictions. Whether the trend is real or putative, it is pronounced enough to make an impression on the medical community. One medical school survey, for example, revealed that 50 percent of the male students and 20 percent of the female students believed that women are more anxious about their bodies than men. And in the seminal research published in 1987 revealing a bias against women in heart disease treatment, Jonathan Tobin, Ph.D., found that, when thallium scans were abnormal, physicians were more likely to attribute women's symptoms than men's to noncardiac causes and that, too often, the cause was presumed to be psychological. In other words, women are more likely to have their symptoms dismissed as "all in their heads" or as psychosomatic.

These presumptions typically play themselves out in experiences like Victoria Mason's. In her mid-forties, Victoria developed a tightness in her throat when she walked against the winter wind. Though Victoria had always been active—she taught jazz dance, and she played golf and tennis—within a couple of years she was too easily winded even for doubles. Yet one doctor after the next failed to screen her for heart disease, and her problem went undetected for twenty years, when she was finally diagnosed and referred for bypass surgery. Women, particularly when they are young, encounter this frustration more than men. It is especially likely to occur when the problem is rare, as coronary heart disease is in forty-five-year-old females.

Ellen Rubino had a similar experience. At twenty-seven, Ellen was healthy, active, physically fit. One evening, shortly after developing a strange, vague sense of doom, Ellen collapsed. By the time the paramedics arrived, Ellen was drenched with sweat, but awake and alert. Her vital signs were normal, and she seemed fully recovered. But she insisted on going to the hospital, where the pattern recurred several times during the next day and a half. The doctors could not ignore the fact that something was wrong, but heart disease never crossed their minds. Perhaps she was suffering from complications of the flu, they conjectured, or maybe she was having seizures. Only when her husband and father insisted that her heart be checked thoroughly did her doctors discover she was suffering from intermittent but severe electrical disruptions.

Like most physicians, those who evaluated Ellen had learned in medical school to tackle diagnosis expediently by looking for what they expected to find. Because of the early reports from the Framingham study (see Chapter 1), they also learned that women rarely get heart disease, and so they never thought to look for it. Even when physicians recognize that heart disease is possible, if the condition is unusually complex or overshadowed by complicating factors, they may miss it. Thus, thirty-two-year-old Jessica Greene saw twelve doctors before she got satisfactory treatment for her palpitations and light-headedness. In the process, one physician after the next shrugged his shoulders and concluded it must be psychosomatic. "One doctor told me all I needed was to go home and get pregnant," Jessica recalled. "When you know you are sick and a physician responds like this, then you develop emotional problems on top of the physical problems."

Another woman with heart trouble agrees. "A string of doctors told me I was having emotional problems until I thought I was going crazy. But when I found a physician to treat me properly, my emotional problems went away."

Dismissing women's complaints as psychosomatic is a convenient way for physicians to reconcile a medical enigma for themselves. Since women's symptoms are often elusive and since research about heart disease in women is scant, their problems can be daunting. Like everyone else, physicians want to be effective, and not being able to resolve their patients' complaints can make them uncomfortable. When patients make insistent demands, physicians sometimes retreat. And when they feel backed into a corner, they may take face-saving recourse. Thus, when a physician concludes that a patient's heart pain is emotional, the conclusion may be a reflection of the physician's frustration or ignorance.

Copping out this way is not reserved for heart disease. In 1862, when French physician Maurice Raynaud first observed the syndrome that bears his name—the circulatory disorder in which fingers and toes suddenly turn cold and blue—he thought the cause was neurosis. He theorized that the condition, which is seen predominantly in women, occurred because emotional distress intensified the body's normal reaction to cold. This explanation held until a physical cause was discovered decades later.

Similarly, migraine headaches, which afflict twice as many women as men, were for years mistakenly attributed to a number of psychological causes, including perfectionism, anxiety, and sexual conflicts. Ultimately, sophisticated understanding of neurochemistry made it clear that in the majority of cases, migraines are triggered by changing levels of hormones.

Having physical problems attributed to emotional causes is not peculiar to women. Before the medical causes of male impotence were demystified, the cause was usually presumed to be psychological.

Whether male or female, with heart disease or another ailment, when a patient is told by a physician, "I can't find anything wrong; the problem must be psychological," the patient is unlikely to identify the failure as the physician's. Women with heart problems, made vulnerable by pain and frustration, typically perceive the physician's conclusion as a reflection of their own inadequacy, as if their symptoms were somehow their fault. Invariably they lose self-confidence, feel frightened, and become angry at the medical profession. At worst, this sequence ends when the patient dies unnecessarily and the cause of death is discovered during an autopsy.

If you have trouble pinning down your diagnosis and getting effective treatment, you must find a different physician. As Lawrence Horowitz, M.D., and author of *Taking Charge of Your Medical Fate*, warns, "Not all doctors are equally skillful. From state to state, from city to city, or hospital to hospital, doctors vary in how well they meet the needs of their patients. There are people in America today who will lose their lives not because of their diseases but because they will choose one doctor's door to open rather than another's. The quality of care in America may vary. The quality of your care doesn't have to."

Women who have endured the frustration, fear, and fury say that with persistence it is possible to find a thorough, caring physician who can not only manage your illness but also restore your confidence in yourself and the medical profession. Jessica Greene ultimately found a thorough and methodical cardiologist who identified her primary disorder as mitral valve prolapse. But because it was obscured by several coexisting conditions, identifying them all and treating them effectively required unusual skill and patience. Feeling very much the veteran of abuse, Jessica advises, "Keep searching until you find the right doctor." Like many other women with similar experience, Jessica also believes that, when you find the right doctor, you'll know it. Jessica knew she was in good hands when her symptoms finally began to subside. Her fear dissipated as well. Another patient echoed Jessica's sentiments: "When I found the right doctor, I wasn't scared anymore. I felt human again."

THE IMPORTANCE OF OPEN COMMUNICATION

When a physician makes a diagnosis and prescribes effective treatment, patient and physician often strike up a relaxed and mutually satisfying partnership, which holds up as long as things go well. But sometimes complications set in and resist resolution. Faced with frustration, the patient can become insistent, the physician can become defensive, and the relationship can deteriorate. Amy Fine faced just this concern. When Amy first developed an abnormally slow heart rate, her cardiologist referred her to a first-rate team of electrophysiologists, who outfitted her with a computer-age pacemaker. Everything was wonderful for three months. Then Amy began to feel the familiar fatigue and dizziness again. Her specialists adjusted the pacemaker to no avail. Solving the problem, they discovered, required replacing the pacemaker and repositioning the leads. Optimistic, Amy submitted to the second surgery, but afterward she felt no better.

Understandably, she was discouraged. Worse, she worried that her physicians would become frustrated and begin to avoid her. Amy, who is a nurse, had seen this pattern more than once, and she addressed the prospect with her physicians head-on. "How long until you guys get frustrated with me and give up?" Amy asked. When they reassured her, Amy was able to put her fear to rest and cope with the ensuing diagnostic struggle. As it turned out, Amy's new problem had nothing to do with her pacemaker but with a viral infection that had occurred coincidentally. She recovered from the infection, her pacemaker is working properly, and Amy is Jazzercising again.

Amy was able to resolve her concerns by communicating candidly with her physicians. Other women have felt compelled to go a step further. Julie Procich, founder of Young Hearts, the new national support group for young adults with heart disease, took charge of her care when treatment threatened to harm her unborn twins. Julie, who has lived with a valve disorder all her life, was five months pregnant when she was hospitalized with endocarditis, a potentially fatal inflammation of the heart. The physician in charge, an infectious disease specialist, recommended a medication that would have left her babies deaf, and Julie refused. She told the doctor she would die before doing anything that would harm her babies, and she arranged a consultation with her cardiologist and obstetrician to find another solution. Three years later, having recovered and given birth to two normal, healthy babies, Julie asserted that patients must exercise their rights and take charge of their care. "We cannot simply take what's told to us as gospel. We must question our physicians and if we know in our hearts that something isn't right, we must refuse to go along with their recommendations."

Furthermore, Julie feels it is the patient's responsibility to compensate for shortcomings of what she calls "diagnosis by the numbers." Unlike physicians of half a century ago, who based their diagnoses on what patients said and the examinations revealed, doctors today rely largely on the results of sophisticated tests. Julie contends, and many other patients agree, that when the patient's experience conflicts with the numbers on the lab report, physicians believe the lab report. "Sometimes," Julie said, "our symptoms are too subtle to show up in the numbers. But we know our bodies better than anybody. We know when we get up in the morning how our hands and feet look.

and when we start to see a difference, we know there is something going on. Never mind what the tests say. We must make the doctor pay attention."

When physician and patient alike feel frustrated or unsure—because the initial diagnosis is perplexing, because the proposed course of treatment is controversial, or because baffling problems arise later on—the best recourse may be a second opinion. Physicians often value the opportunity to share a challenging problem with a respected colleague, if only to get confirmation that their thinking was valid in the first place. At AHI we have weekly meetings just for this purpose. In our "Cath [short for cardiac catheterization] Conferences" we present complex cases and debate the best way to approach them. These presentations always provoke thoughtful discussion and often produce innovative solutions the presenting physician may not have thought of on his or her own. Because second opinions are valuable to patient and physician alike, you should not be embarrassed to ask for one.

MYSTICAL SIGNIFICANCE OF THE HEART

The difficulties that patients encounter as they pursue diagnosis and treatment are understandably frustrating and frightening. Chest pain, palpitations, and difficulty breathing feel threatening. These sensations take on added magnitude because they involve the heart. After all, the heart is, quite literally, the pump of life. And while diseases of other vital organs—the liver and the pancreas, for example—can be just as serious and sometimes more life threatening, heart disease carries unique emotional implications, intensified by the mystical significance the heart traditionally has held.

The heart has occupied a unique position of awe and reverence since the beginning of civilization. In primitive times, cannibals sought strength and courage by eating the hearts of valiant enemies. In ancient Egypt, the mythological god Osiris judged the dead by weighing their hearts. Centuries later, King Edward I of England requested his heart be buried in Jerusalem. The hearts of Byron and Shelley have been preserved. And while David Livingston's body lies in Westminster Abbey, his heart remains in Africa.

Nearly 2,500 years ago, Aristotle argued that from the heart come feeling and emotion, and although we know better today, the metaphor lives on. The heart remains the seat of the soul, and so we speak about sweethearts and broken hearts, soft hearts and cold hearts. We offer heartfelt sympathy, we express our candor in heart-to-heart talks, and, as children, we vowed our sincerity saying, "I cross my heart and hope to die."

Because the heart retains its mystical significance, the implications of heart disease sometimes loom larger than the disease itself, asserts Richard S. Blacher, M.D. professor of psychiatry at Tufts University. Mary Austin, who learned that she had mitral valve prolapse at age forty-four, spoke for many patients when she said, "The heart is almost like a person of its own. Heart disease is so different from any other illness, even cancer." Similarly, Ida Long, who was diagnosed with Prinzmetal's angina, was distraught by the realization that, during her cardiac catheterization, a foreign body touched her heart. "I felt shattered," she said, and reported that it took days to get over the emotional trauma.

Certainly these reactions represent the extreme. Yet, particularly in the context of heart surgery, reverence for the heart and its psychological implications are "staggering," according to Larry Goldman, M.D., and Chase Patterson Kimball, M.D. In *Helping Cardiac Patients*, by Andrew M. Razin and associates, they write, "Beyond its life-sustaining physiological function, the heart performs a central symbolic role in the emotional life as well," and this symbolic role contributes to the unusual and profound emotional responses patients have. Unexplained depression and anxiety frequently occur, as twenty-six-year-old Doris Melbourne found out after an operation to correct a congenital defect. The procedure had gone smoothly and her recovery progressed quickly. By the fourth day after surgery, Doris felt strong enough to wash her hair. But as she bent over the sink and the warm water caressed her head, she suddenly began to sob uncontrollably. To this day, she cannot explain the feelings that prompted this episode or others like it that descended upon her spontaneously over the following three months. Like Doris, many people—and not just women—become childlike, weepy, easily frightened, unusually dependent. These are normal, though not universal, reactions to the physical and emotional upheaval of cardiac crisis.

The emotional ramifications of heart disease can be quite difficult, and having an effective strategy for coping with them can ease the burdens of the experience.

DEALING WITH FEAR OF THE UNKNOWN

Few things are as frightening as the unknown. Thus, Margaret O'Mally, whose experience with mitral valve prolapse appears in Chapter 7, suffered acute anxiety reactions in conjunction with her symptoms until she understood her condition. Her cramps and diarrhea subsided as soon as she realized her disorder wasn't serious, even before beta blockers got her palpitations under control. When we feel threatened, it's human nature to draw catastrophic conclusions, which can be needlessly punitive. For weeks after her heart attack, Sylvia Chester, who would succumb to fatigue without warning or provocation, worried she would never regain her strength; she needed to learn that her weariness was normal and temporary. Similarly, Judith Ralston's brain seemed like a sieve after her valve surgery. She had trouble verbalizing her ideas, frequently lost her train of thought in the midst of a sentence, and had difficulty concentrating and remembering what she read. This seventy-two-year-old woman became convinced she was showing signs of Alzheimer's disease. When she learned that temporary mental disruptions like these are common after heart surgery and that after several months they fade, she had a much easier time managing them.

The first strategy, then, for coping with a crisis or living with a chronic condition is to learn what experiences and emotions you can expect and what they mean. The first stages of recovery after a heart attack or heart surgery are surprisingly rapid and dramatic, but the further along you get in the process, the more slowly recovery progresses. Moreover, recovery from any episode with heart disease is commonly characterized by good days and bad days, rather than steady improvement. Ask your doctor what recovery should be like for you. How long should it take? What kinds of little setbacks are you likely to experience and how should you respond to them? If your condition leaves you with chronic or lingering symptoms, find out what their implications are. Are they dangerous or just annoying? What changes in symptom pattern should you take in stride? What kinds of developments should provoke your concern? If you become troubled, what procedure should you follow to get prompt attention? Fear is pernicious; don't let it fester.

On the contrary, alleviating anxiety can save your life—literally. McGill University researcher Nancy Fraser-Smith demonstrated this when she arranged for nurses to call heart attack patients once a month just to see how they were doing. Whenever a patient sounded apprehensive or had been rehospitalized for any reason, a cardiac nurse visited the patient at home to answer questions, provide information, and, if necessary, make referrals to health care professionals. In this study of five hundred patients, participants in the counseling group received, on average, five or six hours of private counseling over a year's time. This small effort reduced mortality by 50 percent during the year the program was in progress, and four years later the group's survival rate continued to justify the strategy.

SOCIAL SUPPORT

Many women who have recovered from a crisis or learned to live with a chronic condition say they never could have done it without the love and understanding of their husbands, children, and friends. On a practical level, friends and family pitch in with cooking, shopping, and other chores you may not have the energy for. On an emotional level, loving and empathetic people can lift your spirits, help you keep your perspective, offer fresh ideas for solving problems, and keep you from becoming preoccupied with your health. Personal testimony is substantiated by huge population studies that correlate good health to love, friendship, and the commitment of closely knit community.

The converse is also true. Living alone is tied to depression, which in turn has been correlated with increased rates of illness, especially heart attacks. Separate research reveals that loneliness breeds illness and that intense loneliness, particularly in the context of new widowhood, is associated with inordinate rates of depression and death.

Since women are usually older than men when they get coronary heart disease, and since most women outlive their husbands, they are likely to be widowed and living alone by the time they have a cardiac crisis. Some women who live alone have no trouble surrounding themselves with help and companionship. Harriet Silber, the eighty-two-year-old widow whose bypass surgery was mentioned in Chapter 5, credits her swift and smooth recovery largely to the devoted attention of her daughters, who came in from out of town to take care of her. "They were like nurses to me," Harriet said. One stayed for two weeks, the other for five, and by the end of seven weeks, Harriet was comfortable being alone. Eileen Adams, seventy-six, had a comparable experience. Also widowed, she had the constant support and attention of two best friends and neighbors. They brought her food and visited with her every day. When she was ready, they drove her wherever she needed to go.

But sometimes living alone can become a trap, as Mildred Spencer discovered. After Mildred's husband died, she managed alone quite well. At eighty, she had no problems driving, shopping, cooking for herself, and keeping up with the varied necessities of life. She had many friends, her phone was always ringing, and when she felt well, she went out often. But she could never bring herself to ask for favors and she held her friends at arm's length whenever she felt sick.

When Mildred suffered a heart attack, her son and his wife, who live out of town, flew in to be with her, but they could stay only a week. Mildred left the hospital in the care of a hired aide who helped with shopping and cleaning but offered no diversion, no social stimulation, no emotional support. During her convalescence, with its attendant fatigue and discomfort, Mildred became overwhelmed by the ordinarily simple tasks of getting washed and dressed, writing checks, and keeping track of her medical bills. And she had no one to help her keep her perspective. As the weeks went by, she stopped getting dressed and spent the day in her bathrobe. The prospect of going out was daunting. Even her voice began to sound flat and dull.

Alarmed, Mildred's son and his wife flew back for a long weekend. They insisted that Mildred get dressed, and they took her to her favorite restaurant for dinner. They planned some kind of excursion every day, helped Mildred clear her desk, persuaded her to resume contact with her friends, and by the time they left, she was feeling substantially better.

June Pimm, Ph.D., a University of Miami psychologist who has extensively studied social support in the context of depression, believes that widowhood can make women particularly vulnerable to depression, which often stands in the way of complete recovery. Dr. Pimm points to the literature documenting that women, who are more likely to be depressed than men in general, suffer noticeably more than men after heart surgery. One study showed that women who had had bypass had less social support and felt emotionally worse one year after surgery than either male bypass patients or female valve replacement patients. Another study found that women, compared to men, perceived themselves as sicker, less fulfilled, and more depressed.

Widowhood, heart disease, and depression make poor bedfellows.

As Dr. Pimm said, "I am concerned about the research correlating grief to illness and death, and I am particularly worried about widows who have not fully worked through their grief." Her concern seems merited, considering this recent revelation by Duke University's Redford Williams, M.D.: Fifty percent of unmarried patients (compared to 17 percent of those who were married) died within five years after developing heart disease. Close relationships, Dr. Williams found, were the strongest predictor of longevity in the face of heart disease.

Yet women, married or not, seem to have more trouble getting effective, empathetic support than men. "This is a socialization issue, a gender issue, not a heart disease issue," contends David Hall, Ph.D., AHI director of psychological services. "Men tend to be task oriented while women tend to be relationship oriented. Most men have difficulty understanding emotions and expressing feelings. As a result, they have difficulty nurturing."

One woman, describing her husband's discomfort during her convalescence from bypass surgery, said he felt completely inept doing the laundry and taking charge of the kitchen. But those difficulties paled beside the trouble he had as a care giver. This man's hand shook so when he brought his wife her pills, she recalled, that he would spill the water he was carrying.

Another woman, twenty-six years old, woke up one morning with her heart racing at more than one hundred beats a minute, and her husband refused to take off from work or look after the children so she could go to the doctor. She was diagnosed with severe mitral valve prolapse, and as she struggled to get her medication regulated, he worried only about how the wash would get done and the house cleaned. Most men are not as bumbling or callous as these, but many shun the nurturing role nevertheless.

By the same token, many women have inordinate difficulty letting others take care of them. In some cases, the problem stems from an attempt to demonstrate to themselves and the ones they love that heart disease has not upset the family equilibrium, that Mother is still Mother. Some women worry that if they are different, their husbands won't find them attractive and their children, whether young or grown, will pull away from them. In other cases, women have their identity and self-esteem so tied up in their traditional role of caretaker and nurturer that they cannot bear to relinquish it. Regardless of cause, research reveals that following hospitalization for heart disease, women commonly begin dusting, making beds, washing dishes, and doing other chores within days of being discharged. Women who can't or don't keep up with their household tasks commonly feel guilty about their shortcomings and about permitting their husbands, relatives, and friends to help with the housework. Whether actively or passively, many women reject support.

Sometimes, women don't get support because they don't know how to ask for it in a way that men understand. As Deborah Tannen, Ph.D., linguist and author of the best-seller *You Just Don't Understand* explains, men tend to communicate in direct and explicit terms, while women try to influence others through suggestions and innuendoes. Thus, when a woman says, "I think the laundry needs to be done," she might be trying to say, "Please do the laundry," but her husband would be more likely to interpret her statement as an observation than as a request.

When men are reluctant nurturers to begin with and women have trouble communicating their wishes in direct and explicit terms, women can feel abandoned and alone. Forty-three-year-old Carol Vixen's marriage barely survived her chronic arrhythmias because her husband had no capacity for empathy and she did not know how to ask for it. "I had an attack once while we were traveling," Carol remembers, "and being away from home felt really scary. So what does he do? He goes out and leaves me alone. He figured I was safe. He had given me my medicine and helped me into bed, and there was nothing else he could do, so he didn't need to stay around. It never occurred to him that just having him nearby would make me feel more secure. But I couldn't bring myself to say, 'I want you to stay here with me.' Actually, I don't think it ever occurred to me that I had the right to say it."

Because loving attention is so salutary, it pays to think about how you can best benefit from the care your family and friends want to give you. Women who have successfully engineered a support system recommend making direct requests. After surgery, one woman who lives alone made out a schedule for her friends to help with cooking, shopping, and other errands. She managed to have help when she needed it and company when she wanted it. Though she was reluctant to impose at first, she found that her friends appreciated the opportunity to feel useful and got as much out of helping her as she got from their support.

MANAGING TROUBLE AT HOME

Changed Personalities and Strained Relationships

Heart disease can worm its way into people's self-image and change their lives in subtle ways. After valve surgery, thirty-eight-year-old Andrea Winston felt that people viewed her differently, that their eyes seemed to say, "We know you're going to die." Two years later she still interprets the need to take antibiotics before having her teeth cleaned as a symbol of vulnerability. Her operation scar, the anticoagulants she takes daily, and the blood tests she undergoes regularly remind her that heart disease will always be a part of her life. While she believes she is over the worst of her depression, she continues to cry more easily than she used to. She is convinced that heart disease has changed her permanently.

As patient and spouse are transformed by stress and fear, married couples who could once complete each other's unspoken thoughts commonly find themselves talking to apparent strangers. Before her heart attack and bypass surgery, fifty-six-year-old Paula Newman had always been feisty, even combative. Afterward, she was suddenly depressed, weepy, cowering. Her husband was confused by her changed personality. He was also afraid that she might die, worried about how he would endure if she did, angry at her for getting sick and threatening their equilibrium, overwhelmed and resentful at having to take over her household duties, and guilty about his selfish concerns. The feelings that Paula and her husband harbored separately persisted for months and wedged them apart. "Heart disease is like having another child in the house," she said, "but you can't get a baby-sitter and you can't get away."

Anger and resentment acquired a different cast in Carol Vixen's marriage. From the time her two children were toddlers, arrhythmias complicated by asthma kept her bed bound for days at a stretch. She was terrified that she would die, and her husband, whose mother had raised a passel of children without ever needing a nap, berated her for being weak. He made incessant demands, she felt guilty and inadequate for not being able to meet them, and they grew increasingly distant.

Julie Procich, founder of Young Hearts, succinctly says, "Heart disease changes everything." The fear, the anger, the loss of security distort personalities and destroy relationships. Typically, each partner worries silently for fear of overburdening the other. Communication becomes an attempt at mutual mind reading, which is rarely accurate. As neither shares his or her feelings, both withdraw and resentment mounts.

The antidote, says AHI director of psychology David Hall, is open communication. "It's okay to feel bad when things are bad," Dr. Hall advises. He believes that validating fear alleviates fear, and that sharing feelings of frustration and distress can bring couples closer together.

When communication between couples has historically been good, just being instructed to communicate more openly sometimes resolves the problems. Often, however, by the time couples realize they have a problem, it has grown too large for them to solve on their own. If your relationship has become difficult, you might ease the strain by taking your husband with you to support group meetings. Many couples discover that when they hear others reflecting their own problems, solutions become apparent. In addition, many husbands admit that their own ability to empathize improves just by listening to other women who have feelings similar to their wives' and seeing how other husbands cope. Alternatively, consider individual or joint counseling with a mental health professional experienced in the psychological dynamics of medical illness. Short-term therapy can be exceedingly helpful.

Impaired Sexuality

Not surprisingly, cardiac crises can bring sexual intimacy to an abrupt halt. The problem certainly is not universal. Pat Taylor, who had her first heart attack and bypass surgery at age thirty-six, was ready for sex as soon as she was discharged from the hospital. "I asked my doctor when it would be safe for me to make love, and he turned beet red. 'Why are you so red?' I asked him. 'I'm a normal thirty-six-year-old woman.' He just shook his head and said, 'If you can find the way, God bless you.' "

Pat's passion was probably unusual. After heart surgery, many women feel as though they are damaged goods. The scar they see every day serves as a tangible reminder of their vulnerability and can keep them from intimacy. After surgery and heart attacks, many people also find their interest dulled by fear: that they will break their bypasses, dislodge their valves, open their incisions, or cause a heart attack. These fears are natural, but unfounded. Sexual activity cannot damage your surgery, and if you can walk up two flights of stairs without chest pain or shortness of breath, you should have no trouble making love.

Just knowing that sex is safe for your heart should help make it satisfying for you and your partner. It's common, though, for worry to ruin the experience. Ruth Pinna, whose heart attack and angioplasty are mentioned in Chapter 5, was completely preoccupied the first time she had sex after her illness.

"The doctor told me to do it with someone familiar because new partners make sex more stressful. Well, that's fine if you're married or have a steady lover, but what's a single woman like me supposed to do? So here I am with this guy and I'm not sure I even like him, and all I can think about is 'what does he think of my nitro [nitroglycerin] patch,' and 'what if I have a heart attack in the middle?' "

Your first sexual encounters are most likely to be good if they are relaxed and comfortable. Since fatigue can get in the way, choose a time when you feel rested and have time to rest afterward. Since insecurity about yourself and uncertainty about your relationship can also interfere, pick a time when you and your partner feel good about yourselves and each other. If you are worried or frightened, try to share your concerns with your partner. Make the experience romantic. Make it fun. And be patient. You may need a few encouraging encounters before your passion peaks and you can put your fears to rest.

Fear aside, some medication can also interfere with love-making. Although medications pose a more serious problem for men, drugs such as Inderal and Cardizem can dull women's sex drive. If you suspect this problem, mention it to your doctor. Often dosages can be adjusted, prescriptions can be changed, and the problem can be solved.

By far the biggest obstacle to passion arises out of the general emotional turmoil that heart disease creates and the strain it puts on relationships. Julie Procich, whose marriage almost ended during the acute phase of her illness, said, "I was so preoccupied with fear—not of sex but of heart disease—that I couldn't relate to Tom in any way." She added that it took two years before they could hold hands and laugh with abandon. As the threat of her heart disease faded and their relationship returned to normal, her desire also returned.

Carol Vixen, whose husband berated her for being ill, admitted that his coldness brought their sex life to an end. "If someone doesn't empathize with you, the closeness goes. There is no bond, and you have no interest in making love."

In most instances, it's the relationship that needs repair. Sometimes time does the trick. Learning more about your particular kind of heart disease and sharing your experiences in a peer support group (see the section on peer support below) can also help. If problems persist, you might mention them to your doctor, but don't be surprised if he or she feels embarrassed and uncomfortable talking about sex. Sometimes psychotherapy, marriage counseling, or a few sessions with a sex therapist are the best solution.

Helping the Children

When their mother has heart disease, growing children cannot help but be affected. At the very least, their schedule is upset. At worst, they experience a loss of nurturing and feel the very foundation of their security shaken.

AHI director of psychological services David Hall advises that children do best when their lives are disrupted as little as possible. On a practical level, this means going out of your way to keep their activities and routines as familiar and normal as possible. If you are in the hospital and your husband must choose between visiting you and getting your daughter to her weekly karate class, your daughter's karate class should take precedence.

If new child-care arrangements are necessary, try to arrange a one-on-one situation with someone who can provide love as well as care: a close relative, favorite sitter, or good friend. Since children worry about losing their mothers and the love and attention the mother represents, putting your child into a new day-care group would probably feed his fears. Although day care is fine if it is familiar and customary, if it is not, resort to it only if you have no other options.

Children worry most about losing love and nurturing. Often their fears are irrational and can be put to rest with clear, overt, optimistic messages: "Mommy is going to be fine." If you can convey that your love is intact, even in the face of disability, the children should not feel slighted or neglected. Thus, if you can't go upstairs to tuck your son into bed at night, tell him something like, "Mommy can't climb the stairs tonight, so be sure to have Daddy bring you in to the living room so I can give you a hug and kiss good-night."

Despite the best intentions, children respond to the stress and disruption of heart disease, just as adults do. They may have trouble sleeping, begin to act up, or develop problems at school. Be sure your children's teachers know about the health problems at home, and then watch for any dramatic changes in behavior. Should any arise, address them in an investigative, nonjudgmental way. Try approaching the problem with an observation like, "I notice you've been having a lot of bad dreams lately. I'm curious [not concerned, which is a word charged with judgment]; what's wrong?" This kind of approach minimizes criticism and invites the child to express his feelings.

Predictably, the child will respond, "I don't know," or "Nothing's wrong." Then you can begin to suggest some theories. Begin with those that are least threatening: Are you having trouble at school? Is your teacher mean to you? Are you having trouble with the other kids? You may be surprised to discover that something else is going on, and then, of course, you can deal with it. If not, once the conversation is moving freely and comfortably, you can ask, "Are you worried because Mommy is sick?" If the response is yes, you can discuss the child's fears with him. Honest communication is as helpful to children as it is to adults and will give you the opportunity to provide the reassurance that your child needs.

This thumbnail guide is not intended to suggest that children's apprehension is trivial or that it can be relieved by applying a simple formula. If difficulties persist, you might want to consider counseling or family therapy. But women who have had heart disease from the time their children were small commonly feel that their illness has not scarred their children permanently. As one patient put it, "My [teenage] children seem unusually caring and sensitive to my needs and, in general, to the feelings of others. Now, they might have grown up that way regardless, but I like to think that the presence of heart disease in their lives sharpened their antennae a little bit."

PEER SUPPORT GROUPS

Because heart disease can have a far-reaching impact on patients' lives and relationships, many people—sometimes with their spouses—turn to other heart patients for empathy, compassion, and validation of their feelings. "Old friends, even family, don't know what to do with you," complained Paula Newman, who had a heart attack and bypass surgery at fifty-six. "You might look healthy and vital but they know you have been horribly sick, that you still might be horribly sick, and they don't know how to relate to you." Although Paula was surrounded by her friends, her family, and her husband, she felt entirely alone until she met other women with heart disease.

Ellen Rubino, the twenty-seven-year-old whose heart suffered electrical disruptions, put the same feelings another way. "Everyone was nice, but people figured since I was home that everything was just fine. If people don't see a wheelchair or a cast or another symbol of disability, they figure you're okay. But for me the emotional impact was just setting in. Most of my friends didn't want to have to deal with it, so they just carried on their own lives."

Ellen and Paula turned to support groups for empathy and self-esteem. Others, like Andrea Winston, seek reassurance and perspective. "Ever since I had my valve surgery and learned that infection can settle in my heart, I get crazy the second I feel a headache or a scratchy throat," Andrea admitted. But when she calls a friend from the group and hears, "It's normal to get headaches. Everyone gets headaches," it sounds different than it would if her husband gave her the same advice.

Amy Fine sought reassurance of another kind. After two pacemaker operations in a year and the swift recurrence of symptoms, hearing from her physicians that she would be fine didn't carry much weight. But when another woman who had also endured repeated setbacks said, "What you need is a few months of feeling good," Amy felt, for the moment anyway, that she could be patient and optimistic.

Many patients turn to support groups for solid information. Rarely does a physician have enough time to answer all of a patient's questions and resolve all her concerns. Most medical practices do not have nurses or other auxiliary professionals who can meet this need either. The best most of them do is provide an impersonal brochure. By offering regular programs and providing a forum for patients to chat with professionals, support groups fill a serious gap in today's imperfect system of health care.

While support groups are not for everyone, those who embrace them swear by the practical help, information, companionship, and morale boost they provide. If you are interested in finding a group nearby, check with your cardiologist. Some hospitals have groups especially for their patients. There are also a number of national organizations with chapters throughout the country; for example, the American Heart Association has sponsored Mended Hearts for thirty years. To locate a convenient chapter, call your local Heart Association or the national headquarters at (214) 373-6300, or write them at 7320 Greenville Avenue, Dallas, TX 75231. Zipper Clubs, for patients who have had heart surgery, are active in the Northeast: call (215) 887-6644 or write to 1161 Easton Road, Roslyn, PA 19001. The newest addition to these clubs is Young Hearts, which Julie Procich founded in 1990 because she couldn't relate to the "fifty-five-year-old men [she] encountered at Mended Hearts." Young Hearts, intended to meet the unique needs of adults under the age of forty-five, is composed primarily of women. New chapters are sprouting regularly, and for people without a chapter nearby, an effective telephone-newsletter network helps members stay in touch. For more information, write to Young Hearts, P.O. Box 274, Brookfield, IL 60513 or call (708) 387–0918.

CARDIAC REHABILITATION

In many ways, cardiac rehabilitation serves all the functions of support groups with the bonus of promoting physical fitness. Terrified to exert themselves lest they harm their hearts, some patients would be cardiac cripples if not for the reassurance and confidence they acquired in cardiac rehab. These programs help patients increase their stamina and strength, reduce their symptoms, and support their efforts to quit smoking and improve their diet. While studies have shown that, in many instances, patients who exercise at home can achieve the same health benefits as those who attend a formal program, many patients feel that the psychological merits of cardiac rehabilitation are unequaled elsewhere. Some feel that staying in touch with the medical center helps them remain vigilant about their health. Women who might otherwise languish at home find these programs put structure into their day and draw them out. They also help women get into the habit of making exercise a priority in their lives. While women tend to drop out of cardiac rehabilitation for reasons discussed in Chapter 6, those who persist benefit tremendously.

At the age of fifty-seven, four years after Belle Sager had valve surgery, her energy level was so low she couldn't stand without support. Within six weeks of conditioning at AHI she noticed a marked improvement. At the end of twelve weeks she was able to hike two miles in the mountains. That was fifteen years ago. Her medical insurance covers three months of rehab every year, and Belle still takes advantage of every penny's worth.

Rae Harding credits cardiac rehabilitation with restoring her life to normalcy. After emergency bypass surgery in 1988, she never quite recovered. She suffered from shortness of breath, fatigue, and depression. Soon her angina was back, and she had to undergo angioplasty to relieve it. Still, she suffered from shortness of breath. Not now. After two years of ongoing rehabilitation three times a week, which her insurance pays for, this seventy-five-year-old woman feels better than she has in years. She values the social interaction, finds reassurance in the presence of the nurses, and responds to the stimulation of the activity around her. "I give it all I have," Rae said, admitting that, on the days when she is not scheduled for rehab and walks at home, she doesn't feel motivated to walk as fast. Thanks to rehab, Rae has the energy to do all her own housework and enjoy her leisure.

Unfortunately, several studies have documented that, except for high-risk patients, cardiac rehabilitation cannot be credited with saving lives. In other words, patients who do not attend these programs live as long as those who do. Although many patients feel that the greatest benefits of rehabilitation affect quality of life, these benefits are difficult to measure. The studies that discredit rehabilitation base their conclusions on physical outcome alone. In an effort to control costs, some insurance companies have used these studies to avoid paying for rehabilitation unless it is likely to prolong life. If your insurance will not cover your rehabilitation, you might investigate the merits of paying for it yourself.

WHEN PROBLEMS PERSIST

Time, good treatment, and support of various kinds can go a long way to help you adjust to heart disease. Sometimes problems persist nevertheless. Many women claim even though their condition is under control, they continue to experience little problems they have to learn to live with. Sometimes serious complications require ongoing, frustrating medical care, as discussed at the beginning of the chapter. And sometimes emotional problems can endure even in the face of solid recovery.

Some degree of emotional distress is normal for two or three months after a cardiac crisis, and for most people these feelings lift spontaneously. But for some 25 to 30 percent of people, intense, unyielding distress prevents emotional adjustment and threatens their physical well-being. The problems that women have overcoming the emotional impact of heart attacks and heart surgery manifest themselves in the inability to return to work, twisted perceptions of the world around them, distorted body images, permanently strained relationships, and enduring impairment of sexual function. Women who have had a heart attack and who feel anxious, fearful, and dissatisfied with their marriages are especially vulnerable to a second attack, suggests the Recurrent Coronary Prevention Project, the first study of psychosocial complications in women. According to Carl Thorenson, Ph.D., who conducted the study, depression and low self-esteem are at the root of these feelings. Moreover, his analysis showed that depression outweighed diet, cholesterol, and severity of heart disease in predicting which women would die. Since the consequences of major depression can be severe, you would be wise to watch out for it.

Signs of Serious Depression

Depression is an enigmatic entity often, but not always, expressed as intense sadness, dejection, or loss of interest in activities that once seemed enjoyable. Sometimes depression manifests itself solely in physical changes, such as difficulty sleeping, eating, or as a variety of medical symptoms. Because the condition has so many potential faces, the American Psychiatric Association lists nine possible symptoms and defines major depression as the prolonged coexistence of any five:

- a sense of hopelessness and lack of interest in normally stimulating activities
- feelings of apathy or loss of sex drive
- significant change in appetite patterns, often accompanied by noticeable weight loss or weight gain
- change in sleep patterns, either insomnia, disrupted sleep, or increased craving for sleep
- apparent nervous energy or muscle sluggishness
- fatigue or lethargy
- feelings of inadequacy or guilt
- difficulty thinking, concentrating, remembering, or making decisions
- preoccupation with death, expressed death wishes, or thoughts of suicide

During the normal course of your recovery, any combination of these sensations may wax and wane for a few months. Some, like difficulties with concentrating and remembering, may last for six months or more if you have had heart surgery. But if you experience any five of these symptoms concurrently for two weeks without a letup, you should seek professional help. Talk to your cardiologist, who can probably refer you to a therapist qualified to treat this problem. In most instances, short-term therapy is exceedingly successful. Under the right circumstances, short-term treatment with antidepressant medication can work wonders. Professional help can certainly make you feel better and may protect you from future medical catastrophes.

THE RAINBOW AFTER THE RAIN

No one would choose to have heart disease. But for all the pain, fear, and disruption, many people's brush with mortality—whether real or presumed—has made them more appreciative of the life they have. Some have found the motivation to slow down, stop smoking, exercise more. Others claim to have become more mellow and patient. Some make a special effort to nurture their souls. Some say they have grown more sensitive to the needs of others. Having been frustrated by physicians who refuse to listen, they came to realize the importance of being a good listener. Many say heart disease has enabled them to shift their priorities, live for the moment, pursue their dreams. And just about everybody stops to smell the flowers.

Amy Fine shrugged her shoulders and smiled. "So I'm corny. But now I feel the sunshine. I mean I really feel it. I walk through the park and I drink in the scent of the newly cut grass. And when it rains I always look for a rainbow."

TAKE ACTION

Remember these points to protect yourself from unnecessary physical and emotional suffering.

- Don't settle for ineffective medical care. Get a second opinion or change doctors if necessary.
- Make sure you resolve your fears. As questions and concerns arise, jot them down so you don't forget them, and then find

out the best time to talk to your physician. If she seems rushed during your appointment, ask about making an appointment to talk at greater length, either face-to-face or over the telephone. Perhaps your physician has an assistant, a nurse practitioner, or another professional who can talk to you at leisure. Or you can always call the AHI HARTLINE (1-800-345-4278); our professionals will help you in any way they can.

- Avoid isolation and loneliness. Take your family and friends up on their offers of help and companionship. Join a support group. Participate in cardiac rehabilitation. In whatever way feels comfortable, avail yourself of the salutary effects of social support.

- If the emotional distress wears you down, consider getting professional help. Since your illness is bound to affect your husband and children, marriage counseling and family therapy can also be valuable. In most cases, counseling with a member of the clergy, social worker, psychologist, or psychiatrist well versed in the emotional dynamics of physical illness works quickly and effectively. Ask your cardiologist for a recommendation.

CHAPTER 9
The Great Debate: Hormone Replacement Therapy

The facts are clear: Women in their thirties and forties have much less heart disease than men the same age. Women undergo menopause, on average, at age fifty-one. Beginning in their fifties, women experience climbing rates of heart disease. The earlier a woman goes through menopause, the more likely she is to incur heart disease. And the distinctive feature of menopause is loss of estrogen.

The logic is irrefutable. Estrogen, at least the estrogen naturally produced by the ovaries, protects women from heart disease to some extent. Therefore, if postmenopausal women replace the estrogen their ovaries no longer produce, they should sustain the protection of their childbearing years. It's logical, but is it true?

In a word, probably. Some two dozen studies testing whether hormone replacement therapy protects against heart disease have now been completed, and with few exceptions they make a convincing case for taking estrogen. Heart disease aside, the hormone also slows bone loss, which characteristically accelerates after menopause, and cuts in half the risk of brittle, breaking bones, a hallmark of severe osteoporosis.* And estrogen eliminates all the miseries of meno-pause: hot flashes, vaginal dryness, weight gain, facial hair, early wrin-kling, fatigue, and even mood swings. While estrogen's ability to alleviate mood swings has long been implied, the first well-controlled study on this subject, which was published in December 1991, con-firms that estrogen can elevate mood and improve psycholgocial functioning in well-adjusted, healthy women. So why do only a third of America's postmenopausal women take this elixir of youth and well-being?

The answer lies partly in a checkered history that began in 1937, when the *Journal of the American Medical Association* first reported that women are "protected" from heart disease. From the outset, scien-tists presumed the mechanism at work had something to do with blood fats, predominantly cholesterols, and in the 1950s the suspi-cion was verified. Experiments now seen as classic demonstrated that estrogen could prevent the development of atherosclerotic plaque in animals fed a high-fat diet. Then in the early 1970s, in a practice so typical of American medicine, researchers took the next logical step: They tested estrogen on men who had had one heart attack to see if it would protect them from another. While the hormone improved the men's cholesterol levels, it appeared to contribute to a rise in overall mortality, made the men impotent, and provoked heart at-tacks as well as dangerous blood clots in the lungs and legs. Coinci-dentally, in the 1960s, oral contraceptives were developed, and women who took these preparations, especially those who smoked, also became unusually prone to heart attacks and clot-induced strokes. Thus, the consensus arose that estrogen always causes blood clots and is dangerous. To this day, some physicians believe this mis-conception and discourage estrogen use on the basis of it.

The premise on which this conclusion was based is wrong on two accounts. One, it presumed that all estrogen preparations are com-parable, and they are not. Two, it presumed that men and women are physiologically the same, and they are not.

---

* This holds true only for women who do not smoke, according to research published in the *Annals of Internal Medicine* in May 1992. The study concludes that, where bone fractures are concerned, smoking negates the benefits of estrogen. Smokers who take estrogen because they want to protect their bones should give up cigarettes.

ALL ESTROGENS ARE NOT EQUAL: THE LESSON OF ORAL CONTRACEPTIVES

The effect of estrogen on women varies enormously with dose and with the composition of the hormone, as the evolution of oral contraceptives illustrates (see Chapter 3). When birth control pills were first developed, they contained as much as ten times the amount of estrogen used today in either contraceptives or hormone replacement therapy. As oral contraceptives were refined, the estrogen dose was lowered, and risks associated with blood clots diminished. In addition to estrogen, birth control pills contain synthetic progesterone, which, in high dosages, raises LDL, or "bad," cholesterol, lowers HDL, or "good," cholesterol, raises blood pressure, and aggravates diabetes. But when the progesterone dose is low, these problems decrease. Several studies show no increase in heart attacks for women on low-dose pills. The finding is strengthened by an analysis of monkey autopsies that showed that oral contraceptives retarded the development of atherosclerosis. Clearly, the history of oral contraceptives illustrates how different formulations and different dosages of estrogen and progesterone affect the body in complex, widely varying ways.

By the same token, just because estrogens endanger men, there is no reason to automatically conclude that they endanger women. Since men and women respond differently to diagnostic tests, medication, and other kinds of treatment, it is reasonable to expect that women and men react differently to hormones. In fact, study after study suggests that, although supplemental estrogen endangers men, it protects women.

ESTROGEN AS PROTECTION FOR THE HEART

Nearly two dozen studies have evaluated estrogen's ability to protect women's hearts, and the preponderance of evidence suggests that estrogen cuts the risk of heart disease by half. Experts believe that up to half the benefit comes from raising HDL and lowering LDL cholesterols. The remaining 50 percent or more is attributed primarily to estrogen's ability to lower blood pressure and facilitate the metabolism of carbohydrates, thereby decreasing the probability of diabetes. Paradoxically, while large doses of estrogen apparently promote the formation of blood clots, the small doses appropriate for replacement therapy somehow discourage it. In addition, since estrogen receptors have been found in the artery walls and on the heart muscle, experts suspect that estrogen has a direct effect on these tissues. Together these benefits have been credited with protecting women whether they smoke, are obese, or have high cholesterol, high blood pressure, or diabetes. Furthermore, estrogen has prolonged survival in patients who already had serious coronary artery disease and somehow correlates to longer life in general. According to one study of nine thousand older women, those who took estrogen lived longer than those who didn't. The longer they took the hormone, the longer they lived.

The newest and perhaps most convincing evidence was the latest analysis of the women in the Nurses Health Study, which was published in September 1991. Like most studies before it, this one showed that estrogen replacement cut the risk of heart disease in half and that current users (those that use modern formulations of estrogen), as compared to past users, derived the most benefit. The greatest asset of this study is its size: over 48,000 women, more than all the women participating in all other studies combined. Because of the study's size and the excellence of its design, its findings won endorsement from Dr. Claude J. Lenfant, director of the National Heart, Lung, and Blood Institute, and from Dr. Antonio Gotto, chairman of the department of medicine at Baylor College of Medicine and a former president of the American Heart Association.

Contrary to the majority of the research, three small studies show minimal or no benefit, and four studies conclude that estrogen increases risk of heart disease. Of these four, experts agree, only the Framingham research appears significant. However, the Framingham women who developed heart disease were older than those in other studies. They also smoked and took two or three times the estrogen dosage now recommended in the United States. Experts note that the experience of these Framingham women parallels the experience of women who took large-dose birth control pills in the 1960s and 1970s.

William Castelli, M.D., current director of the Framingham study, acknowledges that the "great bulk of evidence" supports the merits of estrogen. He said, "If you weigh all the positives and all the negatives of estrogen replacement therapy, I believe it is beneficial. The estrogen dose should be kept as low as possible, and women should be warned that smokers are asking for trouble."

Elizabeth Barrett-Connor, M.D., an epidemiologist at the University of California, San Diego, and a leading authority on this subject, agrees: "I think the studies are overwhelmingly in favor of estrogen's being beneficial."

PROBLEMS WITH OBSERVATIONAL STUDIES

Of the twenty-two studies conducted, all but one were observational. In other words, researchers gathered a population of women and then asked them about their health and use of estrogen. Observational studies are valuable for the trends they identify and questions they define. But these studies have serious limitations. By relying on the memory of participants, hospital records, or physicians' records, they imply a leap of faith that the information is complete, consistent, and free from bias. In addition, they do not provide baseline data from which to draw comparisons, so there is no way to know how each woman who took estrogen benefited from it. Neither is there any way to know precisely why she took estrogen or how her health compared with the health of those who were never offered the hormone, who were offered it and refused, or who initiated therapy and quit.

By definition, those who stick with a prolonged regimen of estrogen therapy are compliant people. They also tend to exercise regularly, eat intelligently, and practice other healthy habits, and it is difficult to assess the impact of these additional factors. Furthermore, most women who take estrogen replacement are white, well educated, financially comfortable, and lean. In other words, they are already at lower risk before they begin therapy. Because the correlation between health and socioeconomic class is poorly understood, researchers have trouble controlling for these elements.

Parenthetically, the Nurses Health Study, whose findings were applauded in 1991, was minimally affected by the disadvantages of observational research. All the participants in the project were free of heart disease when the study began. The health profiles and medical care of those who took estrogen were unusually similar to those of the women who did not, and the validity of the information on their questionnaires was confirmed by medical records. Nevertheless, even this study leaves a little room for doubt. The only way to prove that these apparent conclusions are valid is with an experiment that begins with women who have never taken estrogen, gives the hormone to half the women, and then compares one group to the other. This kind of data is not yet available.

QUESTIONS SURROUNDING PROGESTERONE

To further confound the dilemma, virtually all the research to date on estrogen replacement therapy looks at the impact of estrogen alone. But in the 1970s, disproportionately large numbers of women who took estrogen without progesterone developed cancer of the uterus; the estrogen they took caused a steady buildup of the uterine lining, called the *endometrium*, which was never shed as it is during the normal menstrual cycle. To prevent endometrial cancer, women began taking progesterone as well. The progesterone causes the endometrial lining to slough off and thus prevents cancer of the uterus. But as experience with oral contraceptives illustrates, in large doses progesterone can lower HDL, raise LDL, and thereby offset 25 to 50 percent of estrogen's cardiac protection.

What about small doses? Like large doses, small doses also protect the uterus. Unlike large doses, however, small doses of progesterone may actually protect the heart. While the evidence so far is scarce, several discoveries suggest this possibility. One, some low-dose progesterones used in oral contraceptives caused a drop in LDL cholesterol, although they were associated with a slight increase in triglycerides. Two, in the 1989 Rancho Bernardo study, women taking estrogen and progesterone together had lower triglyceride counts and blood pressure than women taking estrogen alone. More important, although their cholesterol profile was not quite as good as that of those taking "unopposed" estrogen (without progesterone), it was substantially better than the profile of those taking no supplements and "remarkably similar" to that of those taking estrogen alone. Three, animal research reported in 1990 suggested that estrogen and very small doses of progesterone might control heart disease more effectively than estrogen alone. Curiously, the study showed that the baboons given just estrogen had better cholesterol profiles, but those on combination therapy developed fewer plaque deposits in their arteries. The researchers suspect that their findings reflect one of the complex and mystifying interactions of estrogen and progesterone. Four, researchers at the Society for Epidemiologic Research reported in June 1991 that, in a controlled experiment of women, those on combination therapy had a healthier cholesterol profile than those on estrogen alone. This is a very important finding, contends Charles Hennekens, M.D., one of the principal investigators of the Nurses Health Study. "It may lead us to the conclusion that combined preparations are actually better than unopposed estrogen."

Before any firm conclusions can be drawn, large clinical experiments must methodically test the various protocols. After baseline data has been gathered, the women must be randomly assigned either estrogen alone, estrogen combined with progesterone, or a placebo. Then they must be monitored periodically to obtain the data necessary for valid comparisons. And to protect the results from bias, participants must be evaluated by professionals who have no knowledge of what drug the women are taking.

THE PEPI STUDY

The first study to evaluate estrogen and progesterone replacement systematically got under way in 1991. The Postmenopausal Estrogen/ Progestin Interventions Trial (PEPI) is evaluating 875 menopausal women aged forty-five to sixty-four for three years. Before the trial began, participants had a mammogram, an endometrial biopsy, a bone density scan, and comprehensive blood tests to analyze their cholesterol and its fractions, blood pressure, insulin, and level of fibrinogen, a blood-clotting element that helps to predict the likelihood of stroke and heart attack. These tests are being repeated several times during the study. When it is over, PEPI will show how estrogen alone and estrogen combined with progesterone in a variety of doses and regimens affect cardiac risk factors over a three-year period.

The trial will also begin to fill the gaping abyss of ignorance surrounding the workings of a healthy middle-aged woman's body. The bone-density studies will help to clarify the normal distribution of bone mass, which may be different from distributions in women highly susceptible to osteoporosis. By tracking such indicators as levels of depression, overall health status, symptoms of menopause, and sexual function and satisfaction the study will assess the impact of menopause and replacement hormones on quality of life. Finally, the endometrial biopsies may provide some clues to the way unopposed estrogen influences uterine cell changes. Researchers suspect that the cancer induced by estrogen therapy is more localized and less virulent than uterine cancer of other kinds, and the biopsies may help to clarify whether the affected cells are actually different. Alternatively, since women on estrogen replacement get regular medical care, their endometrial cancer may just appear milder because it is detected and treated early. For all the information PEPI will provide, it will not resolve every concern about hormone replacement with certainty.

What will PEPI tell for sure? "That women eagerly respond to a call for volunteering and random allocation," answered Irma Mebane, Ph.D., project coordinator for the National Institutes of Health. As the Framingham study taught us more than thirty years ago, study results must be verified and reverified before they can be trusted.

Moreover, because PEPI runs only three years, it will not confirm whether hormone replacement therapy prevents heart attacks and strokes. Despite the periodic cancer and osteoporosis screenings, the study will not yield comprehensive information on these diseases. Beyond early cell changes, it will tell little about endometrial cancer. As for osteoporosis, we know that estrogen is the single most reliable method for saving bone and that bone loss is accelerated during the early years of menopause. But how much bone must we preserve to prevent fractures twenty or thirty years down the line? How thin do bones have to be at the start of menopause to define certain risk? PEPI will not answer questions like these.

And then there is the most disturbing concern of all: breast cancer.

THE THREAT OF BREAST CANCER

Few diseases elicit more fear than breast cancer. As magazines, movies, and models regularly remind us, the breast is a Western icon of sexuality. Breast cancer is synonymous with pain, disfigurement, and death. While heart disease can be every bit as demoralizing and debilitating, breast cancer is feared more and perceived as worse. And there is good reason to suspect that estrogen may endanger breast health.

The breasts of all mammals contain estrogen receptors, and when lab animals are given a small amount of estrogen, they develop breast cancer. Women exposed to little natural estrogen, either because they begin menstruating late or because they have an early natural or surgical menopause, have a reduced risk of breast cancer. In addition, antiestrogen therapy is one of the leading treatments for some kinds of breast cancer.

But the indictment against estrogen's causing breast cancer is mostly circumstantial. The largest single American study to address the question was the Nurses Health Study. The report, issued in 1990, found that women who take estrogen for ten years incur a 30 to 40 percent increase in their risk of breast cancer. While this sounds enormous, it amounts to about half the risk a woman faces if her mother had breast cancer.

The most incriminating evidence against hormone therapy comes out of Europe, but for the most part, the hormone formulations used in America are different. Women in the European studies took synthetic estrogen. These manufactured estrogens are far more potent than the natural compounds used almost exclusively for postmenopausal therapy in the United States. Here, 75 percent of estrogen selected for postmenopausal treatment is Premarin, conjugated estrogen derived from the urine of pregnant horses (hence the mar[e] in Premarin)—not a particularly appealing thought, but apparently a safer compound.

In 1989, a highly publicized Swedish report showed that therapy combining progesterone and synthetic estrogen raised a woman's risk of breast cancer fourfold, but the number of subjects in the study was tiny. Other studies of combined therapy are mixed; some show that progestin impedes the development of cancer.

In an effort to make sense out of the conflicting data, epidemiologists subjected sixteen comparable studies to a single statistical analysis. This meta-analysis revealed that women who took estrogen for less than ten years incurred virtually no risk, and that when women stopped taking the hormone, their risk declined. More important, it showed that using estrogen for fifteen years increased risk of breast cancer by 30 percent and that women with a family history of breast cancer incurred a substantially higher risk. However, those who took estrogen longest had begun their therapy when dosages were larger than those used today. Especially since the effect of estrogen varies so widely with dosage, it is difficult to interpret these results in terms of the small dosages prescribed now.

Moreover, meta-analysis is a controversial tool. By pooling studies, the analysts deal in large numbers, which presumably give their results greater statistical clout. But pooling studies muddies the impact of each contributing factor. In this meta-analysis, the women took varying forms, dosages, and combinations of hormones. Some of the women began therapy before menopause. Consequently, it is difficult to know what the conclusions mean.

So far the data on risk boil down to much the same bottom line as the data on benefit: probable but not proven. At this point, most experts agree to equivocate. Dr. Elizabeth Barrett-Connor, who believes that the benefits of estrogen outweigh the risks, says, "We have to worry about breast cancer." Nanette Wenger, M.D., a renowned authority on cardiology, talks about a "possible" risk for breast cancer. Charles Hennekens, M.D., one of the principal investigators of the Nurses Health Study, speaks about the "possibility of slight increased risk with long duration of use." Most experts agree that estrogen will not cause new tumors but that, in susceptible women, prolonged use may cause potential tumors to flourish. On balance, benefits are greater than risks, but the risks are real.

WEIGHING THE PROS AND THE CONS

In 1989, Diana Petitti, M.D., M.P.H., University of California epidemiologist, felt there was no scientific basis for recommending estrogen, period. "I'm conservative about these things," she said at the time. "I think people shouldn't take drugs without very clear benefits. Other people take the opposite view. Both may be reasonable, but neither is scientific."

Although Dr. Petitti's philosophy has not changed, her opinion about estrogen therapy has. Today she says, "The evidence supporting protection of the heart is quite strong," and she recommends that women seriously consider taking estrogen if their risk of heart disease is high. However, she adds, the effect of progesterone remains a mystery and anyone who decides to take estrogen primarily to prevent coronary heart disease cannot, on the basis of available research, justify taking progesterone.

The National Women's Health Network (NWHN), a national organization devoted solely to women and health, takes a more conservative position still. In its position paper on hormone replacement therapy published in 1989 the NWHN asserted, "We are critical of the routine prescribing of hormones for healthy women because of the known risks associated with the drugs used and the lack of complete data on risks and benefits." Since estrogen therapy has been proven to protect against heart disease when women have lost their ovaries prematurely through surgery, the NWHN endorses estrogen for women whose ovaries have been removed during their childbearing years. The NWHN also accepts the idea of estrogen therapy for those who experience extreme menopausal discomforts or are particularly susceptible to osteoporosis.

While a look-before-you-leap attitude is certainly warranted, too often the voice of restraint is tinged with troubling hostility. "We object to the view of normal menopause as a deficiency disease. Menopause does not automatically require treatment," the NWHN contends. Similarly, a 1989 *Ms.* magazine article entitled "The Estrogen Fix" begins, "It's difficult to fathom medicine's love affair with estrogen." Author Andrea Boroff Eagan continues, "Consideration of estrogen, its benefits, and risks, raises more than just medical and scientific questions, however; it speaks directly to medicine's view of women, or the deeply held belief that aging is somehow incompatible with 'health and femininity.' " Statements like these imply that estrogen treatment is somewhat akin to sabotage, and one must question advice that is rooted in hostile suspicion.

Many women who reject hormone therapy operate more on the basis of emotion than reason. They object to its inherent artificiality and they recoil at the prospect of "taking medicine." Conversely, many of those who embrace hormones are equally drive by passion. Afraid of aging, they do in fact seek a youth potion and choose to ignore insistent questions about risk. Whether pro or con, most women bring strong feelings to this subject.

Sentiment is intensified by the reactions, both positive and negative, that women have had to taking the drugs. Some women cannot tolerate the monthly bleeding caused by some progesterone regimens used in combination therapy. In addition, many women find the following side effects intolerable: breast engorgement and tenderness, headaches, nausea, uterine cramps, and bloating. Sometimes hormones induce the same three symptoms of menopause they are prescribed to prevent: weight gain, depression, and mood swings. When begun long after menopause, therapy can cause breast nodules and blood clots in the legs. As with any drug, adjusting the dosage often eliminates the problems, but many women prefer to abandon therapy. In contrast, thousands of women experience virtually no negative side effects and love what their hormones do for them. They find that replacement therapy makes their skin softer and smoother, gives them more energy, lubricates their vaginas, and makes them more responsive sexually. Many say that, although their breasts are tender at first, the tenderness goes away after six months or a year. These women feel threatened by the mere thought of relinquishing their hormones.

At this point the data are conflicting and incomplete, and it will be many years before all the questions are answered. In the meantime, the available research boils down to this: Estrogen absolutely does protect the heart when women have lost their ovaries prematurely and probably reduces the risk of heart attack and stroke in all postmenopausal women. Estrogen, together with sufficient calcium consumption and weight-bearing exercise (see Chapter 10), is also the best way to prevent or delay osteoporosis and is credited with reducing fractures by half. And it is the best treatment for the discomforts of menopause. But estrogen alone increases the risk of uterine cancer. If you add progesterone, you eliminate that risk, but you may decrease the protection that estrogen affords your heart. And if you are susceptible to breast cancer, hormone therapy may increase your risk slightly.

Epidemiologically speaking, among any two thousand postmenopausal women in any given year, twenty will get heart disease and twelve will die of it. Six will develop breast cancer and two will die of it. Three will develop uterine cancer, and one will die of it. Eleven will suffer fractures because of osteoporosis. Among those who break a hip, only half will ever recover fully, and as many as one in five will die of complications within a year. These statistics suggest that, for the population at large, more lives can be saved with hormone replacement therapy than lost because of it. This conclusion was verified by a 1991 University of California study showing that women who take estrogen live longer than those who do not. Those who used estrogen had death rates 20 percent below those who never did. Women who took estrogen for at least fifteen years had death rates 40 percent below nonusers. In other words, the longer women took the hormones, the longer they lived. This study shows that the protection against heart disease and osteoporosis outweighs the risks of breast and uterine cancer. Moreover, the disparity among risks is so great that a woman vulnerable to both cancer and heart disease might be better off taking estrogen than not.

Consider, for example, the dilemma of forty-six-year-old Alice Jefferson. As a child, Alice had rheumatic fever that led to valve replacement surgery in 1987. Within three years, however, she was suffering from fatigue and congestive heart failure. Her heart had deteriorated to the point where fluid was collecting in her lungs and activities like vacuuming made her heart race, brought on blurred vision, and left her gasping.

Even if Alice were not otherwise susceptible to coronary heart disease, her heart dysfunction would jeopardize her heart muscle; contracting inefficiently, it sends a diminished supply of blood into the circulatory system and thus limits the amount that can reach her coronary arteries. In addition, her sister and her father both have heart disease, Alice's cholesterol and blood pressure are high, and she smokes. Finally, Alice had her ovaries surgically removed when she was thirty-three and never took replacement estrogen. This early loss of estrogen put her at even greater risk for coronary heart disease. Alice would be a prime candidate for estrogen replacement, but her mother and sister both have breast cancer.

Traditionally, Alice's family history of breast cancer would preclude her from taking estrogen. But statistically speaking, estrogen stands to protect her health more than endanger it, despite her mother's and sister's breast disease. In addition to lowering Alice's cholesterol and blood pressure, estrogen would probably boost Alice's energy level and help her achieve an overall feeling of well-being. Consequently, a responsible and prudent physician just might take this tack: First, learn whether the mother's and sister's breast cancers feed on estrogen. Some do; others do not. This information should be in the mother's and sister's medical records. Second, schedule Alice for a mammogram. If the family's cancers were not estrogen-dependent, if Alice's mammogram was clean, and if Alice agreed to continue having mammograms every six months, estrogen therapy might well be a viable option for her.

SHOULD YOU OR SHOULDN'T YOU?

Should You Take Hormones?

Experts agree that hormone replacement therapy is not for everyone. Whether it is good for you is a decision you must make with your physician based on your individual preference, symptoms, medical history, and risk profile. Current medical wisdom suggests that women over sixty-five should not begin therapy because there is no research for reference. In addition, certain medical conditions make hormone replacement dangerous: a history of blood vessel disease, such as phlebitis; breast, uterine, or ovarian cancer; and gallbladder, liver, or kidney disease. If you cannot or do not want to take hormones, there are other other ways to prevent heart disease and osteoporosis (see Chapter 10).

What Is Your Reason for Taking Estrogen?

By understanding what your goal is in taking hormones, you and your doctor can make the best choice of formulation and dosage.

If preventing heart disease is your aim, studies suggest that 0.625 milligrams of Premarin can lower your risk at least 50 percent, which, to quote Elizabeth Barrett-Connor, is "remarkable protection." Studies show that current users derive greater benefit than past users regardless of how long they once took estrogen. For most women, 0.625 milligrams is a large enough dose to raise HDL 10 to 14 percent and lower LDL 4 to 8 percent. At the same time, this dosage is small enough not to induce blood clots. By taking the medication orally, you assure that, before it gets into your bloodstream, it passes through the liver, where it appears to have its greatest impact on lowering cholesterol. Many physicians prescribe estrogen for twenty-five days followed by a lapse of five days in an attempt to mimic the estrogen curve of the normal menstrual cycle. However, a growing number of physicians believe that, since the ovaries produce estrogen continuously, it is better to take estrogen every day, and there is no research to indicate otherwise. Participants in the PEPI trial selected to receive estrogen will take 0.625 milligrams of Premarin daily, with no five-day lapse.

Perhaps you stand a greater risk of developing osteoporosis. Light-skinned, small-boned, slim women are particularly at risk. A family history of osteoporosis or hip fractures, sedentary life-style, low intake of calcium, a history of certain illnesses such as hyperthyroidism or kidney disease, alcohol use, and cigarette smoking also contribute. In addition, young women with known estrogen deficiency, or women who stopped menstruating because of eating disorders or excessive exercise are also vulnerable. Investigators are finding that estrogen-deficient women in their twenties and thirties are losing substantial bone mass. Studies show that bone loss is particularly severe in the first few years of menopause and when women cease taking estrogen. Therefore, if you choose to take estrogen, you should begin taking it as soon as you go through menopause and plan to take it indefinitely.

IS ESTROGEN THERAPY FOR YOU?

YES, IF YOU	NO, IF YOU
have high cholesterol, high blood pressure, or are otherwise at risk for coronary heart disease	have had a heart attack or stroke recently
are susceptible to osteoporosis	have a history of phlebitis or a tendency to abnormal blood clotting
suffer from the symptoms of menopause	have liver or kidney disease
	have a history of breast or uterine cancer
	are pregnant

Estrogen can be taken through the skin via a medicated patch as well as by mouth. These patches look like Band-Aids and work the same way as nitroglycerin patches, which control chest pain, or scopolamine patches, which control seasickness. "Transderm" or skin patches, as they are called, permit the medication to be absorbed into the bloodstream directly through the skin, without passing through the intestinal tract. Since transderm estrogen does not pass through the liver, where it has its greatest impact on cholesterol levels, it does not protect the heart as well as oral estrogen. However, the patch and the pill are comparable in their ability to help prevent osteoporosis.

If your primary concern is reducing menopausal symptoms, either the patch or the pill will work. Many women find they can wean themselves off estrogen after about five years. This is something you and your doctor should work out together.

Should You Take Progesterone?

If your uterus has been removed surgically, you don't need progesterone. If your uterus is intact, however, progesterone can protect you from uterine cancer. However, if your goal is to protect against heart disease, taking progesterone may be counterproductive. Since

COMMON SIDE EFFECTS

Estrogen	changes in vaginal bleeding pattern
	tender, engorged breasts
	nausea, vomiting, abdominal cramps
	bloating and weight gain
	headaches and dizziness
	depression
	fatigue
Estrogen and progesterone combination	rise in blood pressure in susceptible people
	premenstrual-like syndrome
	changes in libido
	changes in appetite
	bladder inflammations
	mood swings
	headache, dizziness, fatigue
	backache

there are insufficient data, some experts—including Dr. Charles Hennekens and Dr. Diana Petitti—do not recommend combined therapy at this time. For women who have had a hysterectomy, this position poses no threat. For everyone else, however, it presents a real dilemma. One solution: Take estrogen alone and have annual endometrial biopsies just to make sure that uterine cancer is not developing. "I don't want to trivialize endometrial cancer. But the truth is, it is neither a common nor a highly fatal cancer. So taking unopposed estrogen and having periodic biopsies would be a reasonable decision," said Dr. Petitti.

In contrast to Drs. Hennekens and Petitti, other experts feel it is better to take progesterone and protect the uterus even if the protection from heart disease is compromised. When progesterone is recommended, it is usually prescribed in one of two protocols:

- 5 or 10 milligrams of Provera taken for ten to fourteen days. These dosages will protect the uterus but may cause monthly bleeding. These dosages are also small enough to prevent mood swings for most women.
- 2.5 milligrams of Provera daily. This protocol induces intermittent, unpredictable bleeding for as little as six and as long as eighteen months. Under this protocol, the endometrium ultimately atrophies, and then bleeding ceases forever. Women who can put up with the initial unpredictable bleeding like the idea of ultimately never getting their periods again. In addition, the smaller dose of Provera tends to cause fewer side effects and seems to be more consistent with cardiac protection than the larger dose.

The PEPI study is comparing several progesterone regimens: 2.5 milligrams of Provera daily; 10 milligrams of Provera for twelve days a month, and 200 milligrams of a different progestin for twelve days a month.

TAKE ACTION

If you take hormone therapy, monitor changes in your body as you would with any drug. If side effects become troublesome, work with your doctor to modify the dosage and arrive at a regimen that is as comfortable as it is beneficial.

Since estrogen might accelerate the growth of some breast cancers, you must be particularly vigilant about your breasts. Be sure to examine your breasts once a month and have mammograms at least every other year until you reach age fifty and yearly after that.

Ask your doctor about signs of trouble and report any abnormal vaginal bleeding at once.

CHAPTER 10

Take Action to Protect Your Health: The Diethrich Program

No one can live forever. Scientists estimate that if all cancer and heart disease were eliminated, the average life expectancy would increase only about three years. So why bother with clean living when hedonism is so much more fun? Because we're not talking about an "average life"; we're talking about your life. Because, if you eat healthfully, exercise moderately, use medication prudently, don't smoke, and keep your stress in check, you stand the best chance of living your last years vigorously and independently.

We all have the power to take charge of our life-style. By looking after ourselves and getting good medical care, we can delay disability for as long as fifteen years, scientists estimate. Although genes and other factors beyond our control sometimes thwart our best efforts, to a great extent we can improve our health just by making the commitment to take care of ourselves. What's more, it's never too late to start. Research conclusively proves that healthful habits can postpone or prevent a first heart attack by slowing the atherosclerotic process. But even if you have already had a heart attack, or two or three or more, you can forestall future attacks by reducing your risks.

This is the premise of the Diethrich Program, an eight-week protocol including comprehensive cardiac evaluation, nutritional guidance, personalized exercise prescription, psychological support, and stress management. Inspired by such successful plans as Pritikin's, the Diethrich Program was designed in 1980 specifically for patients disabled by heart disease but for whom surgery or angioplasty was not an option. The patients who enter our program suffer an average of eight episodes of angina a week. By the end of two months on the program they average less than one episode a week, they're more active, and they need less medication. In addition, our patients lose about two pounds a week and demonstrate impressive reductions in cholesterol and triglycerides.

We devised the Diethrich Program in 1980 for thirty-eight-year-old Pat Taylor, whose two heart attacks and two failed attempts at bypass surgery had left her crippled with chest pain. When she first came to AHI, she could not climb stairs or walk fifty feet. By the end of eight weeks in the Diethrich Program, she had lost fifteen pounds, had lowered her cholesterol 10 percent, could walk on the treadmill for ten minutes without pain, and had been weaned from her seven heart medications. Over the ensuing months she lost more weight, lowered her cholesterol further, maintained her exercise regime, and remained symptom free. Six years later, angiography showed that her atherosclerosis had been halted. At this writing, she is still feeling good physically and emotionally.

Pat and her many peers who have walked the treadmill in the AHI conditioning center are proof that the Diethrich Program, whose components form the basis of this chapter, works as both treatment and a preventive measure. Moreover, research implies that women can gain more from heart-smart living than men. Dean Ornish, M.D., whose landmark study demonstrated how a very low-fat diet, regular exercise, and reducing stress could shrink plaque in the coronary arteries, found that women had more impressive results than men. Other studies showed that when women and men are exposed to the same high-fat diets, stressful conditions, and other risk factors, men succumb to heart disease more readily than women. Most recently, angiographic analyses of men and women with comparable risk profiles revealed that coronary artery disease progresses more slowly in women than in men. Together, this research implies that women are inherently more resistant to heart disease than men and that preventive strategies should benefit them more. Considering how heart disease disables women, the prospect of turning disease around or at least slowing it down is indeed alluring.

HOW TO EAT SMART

Limiting Fats and Cholesterol

If you followed a traditional Chinese diet—the one Chinese peasants eat, not the deep-fried take-out fare in America—you probably wouldn't have heart disease or, for that matter, diabetes, osteoporosis, breast cancer, or colon cancer. You could probably also eat as much as you want and still be thin; the Chinese eat one-fifth again as much as we do but are 25 percent leaner. The secret? Scant fat. In 1990, a huge epidemiological study designed by Cornell University's T. Colin Campbell, Ph.D., comparing the typical Chinese diet to ours, showed that the Chinese eat approximately one-third less fat, double the carbohydrates, and a tenth the animal protein we do. Although they consume minuscule amounts of red meat, they do not suffer from anemia. And although they consume virtually no dairy products, they do not suffer from osteoporosis. Moreover, once the Chinese adopt Western eating habits, they acquire our diseases of affluence, so their Asian genes apparently cannot be credited with protecting them.

Convincing by itself, the Chinese study supports an impressive body of research documenting the merits of a low-fat diet. Patients in the Diethrich Program have consistently shown that a low-fat diet, together with other components of the protocol, lowers LDL cholesterol and improves the ratio of total cholesterol to HDL. Dr. Dean Ornish proved with angiography that this formula for living not only helps patients feel better but can actually shrink blockages in their coronary arteries. The Framingham research showed that cutting back on fat can reduce cholesterol levels 10 percent or more.

The fat we eat influences the cholesterol in our blood and thus affects heart disease directly. A high-fat diet also affects heart disease indirectly by promoting obesity. Gram for gram, fat holds more calories than carbohydrates. Moreover, because of differences in the ways different foods are metabolized, the fats we eat tend to pad our waists and hips while other types of food are more likely to be burned off for energy. Consequently, a high-fat diet tends to make us fat, and, as Framingham, the Nurses Health Study, and numerous other research concludes, the farther women's weight climbs above normal, the more vulnerable they become to high blood pressure and diabetes, both risk factors for heart disease. The converse is also true. If you are overweight and go on a very low fat diet, you will probably lose weight. In so doing, you will lower your blood pressure, raise your HDL, and, if you have Type II diabetes, probably bring it under control.

Although some experts have worried that reducing fat intake markedly would compromise women's HDL advantage, this concern appears not to be valid. According to two studies published in the journal *Circulation* late in 1991 (one by Dr. Margo A. Denke and Dr. Scott Grundy at the University of Texas, the other by Sidika Kassim and associates at Wayne State University), a marked reduction in fat consumption led to substantial drops in total and LDL cholesterols, but insignificant changes in "good" HDL.

Separate from heart disease, reducing fat consumption appears to benefit the immune system and helps prevent several cancers. A University of Massachusetts study showed that a 9 percent reduction in fat (from 32 percent to 23 percent of one's total daily calorie consumption) produced a 50 percent increase in natural killer cells, a type of white blood cell that destroys viruses and developing tumors. While the evidence linking low-fat diets to cancer prevention is not yet conclusive, verification is mounting. Red meat is the chief culprit in colon cancer, says the Nurses Health Study. Women who ate a main dish of beef, pork, or lamb every day developed colon cancer at two and a half times the rate of those who indulged less than once a month. Fat intake also appears to be correlated with hormones that trigger cancer of the ovaries, uterus, and breast. Diets high in animal protein, which are by definition high in fat, promote growth in children and make girls menstruate early; early menstruation is correlated to breast cancer. In China, by comparison, where diet contains half the fat as in the American diet, women rarely begin to menstruate before age fifteen, and they have only one-fifth the rate of breast cancer. And in Japan, where diet is rapidly becoming Westernized, breast cancer incidence is rising dramatically, as are cases of heart disease and cancers of the ovaries and uterus. Considering the possible connection between estrogen replacement and breast cancer, a low-fat diet is particularly important for women taking hormone replacement therapy.

How low is low? Americans typically consume a diet composed of 35 to 42 percent fat, nearly half of which comes from meat, dairy, and saturated vegetable fats. In contrast, the American Heart Association and the Surgeon General's nutrition guidelines recommend a maxi-

Proportion of Monounsaturated, Polyunsaturated, and Saturated Fats in Various Dietary Fats

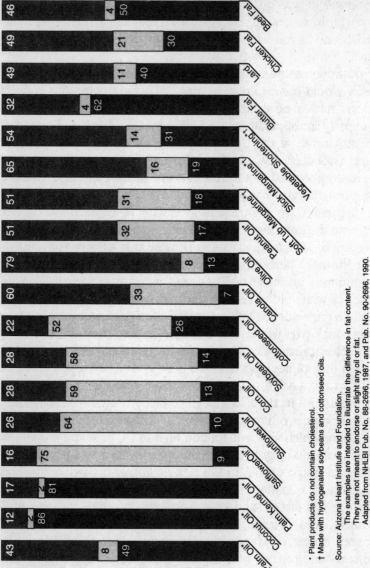

Percentage of Fat Type

■ % Monounsaturated Fat
▨ % Polyunsaturated Fat
■ % Saturated Fat

Fat	Mono	Poly	Sat
Beef Fat	46	4	50
Chicken Fat	49	21	30
Lard	49	11	40
Butter Fat	32	4	62
Vegetable Shortening†	54	14	31
Stick Margarine†	65	16	19
Soft Tub Margarine†	51	31	18
Peanut Oil*	51	32	17
Olive Oil*	79	8	13
Canola Oil*	60	33	7
Cottonseed Oil*	22	52	26
Soybean Oil*	28	58	14
Corn Oil*	28	59	13
Sunflower Oil*	26	64	10
Safflower Oil*	16	75	9
Palm Kernel Oil*	17	2	81
Coconut Oil*	12	2	86
Palm Oil*	43	8	49

* Plant products do not contain cholesterol.
† Made with hydrogenated soybeans and cottonseed oils.

Source: Arizona Heart Institute and Foundation.
The examples are intended to illustrate the difference in fat content.
They are not meant to endorse or slight any oil or fat.
Adapted from NHLBI Pub. No. 88-2696, 1987, and Pub. No. 90-2696, 1990.

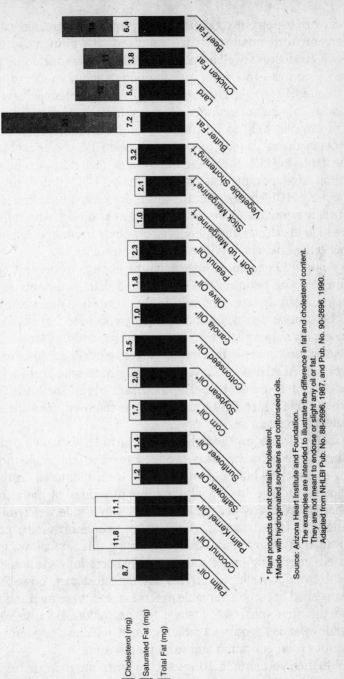

Actual Amount of Fat and Cholesterol in One Tablespoon of Various Dietary Fats

Beef Fat — 14, 6.4
Chicken Fat — 11, 3.8
Lard — 12, 5.0
Butter Fat — 31, 7.2
Vegetable Shortening† — 3.2
Stick Margarine† — 2.1
Soft Tub Margarine† — 1.0
Peanut Oil* — 2.3
Olive Oil* — 1.8
Canola Oil* — 1.0
Cottonseed Oil* — 3.5
Soybean Oil* — 2.0
Corn Oil* — 1.7
Sunflower Oil* — 1.4
Safflower Oil* — 1.2
Palm Kernel Oil* — 11.1
Coconut Oil* — 11.8
Palm Oil* — 8.7

Cholesterol (mg)
Saturated Fat (mg)
Total Fat (mg)

* Plant products do not contain cholesterol.
†Made with hydrogenated soybeans and cottonseed oils.

Source: Arizona Heart Institute and Foundation.
    The examples are intended to illustrate the difference in fat and cholesterol content.
    They are not meant to endorse or slight any oil or fat.
    Adapted from NHLBI Pub. No. 88-2696, 1987, and Pub. No. 90-2696, 1990.

mum of 30 percent total fat, 10 percent from saturated fat and 20 percent from unsaturated fat. Saturated fat—from meat, fish, and dairy products as well as from vegetable sources including palm oil and coconuts—interferes with the body's ability to eliminate excess cholesterol and, like cholesterol itself, raises cholesterol levels in the blood. Polyunsaturated fats, such as safflower, corn, sunflower, and soybean oils, help to rid the body of excess cholesterol. But in the process, these fats tend to lower the good HDL cholesterol as well as the damaging LDL cholesterol. Monounsaturated fats, including olive, canola, and peanut oils, appear to lower LDL cholesterol without touching HDL cholesterol. However, even monounsaturated fats are partially saturated. Olive oil is 13 percent saturated. And since all fats are high in calories and therefore contribute to obesity, the healthiest diet is the one which is lowest in all forms of fat.

While a 30-percent-fat diet might be enough to prevent heart disease in some people, Dr. Ornish found that, in patients already afflicted, heart disease continued to progress when patients followed a 30 percent-fat diet. Studies consistently conclude that healthy eating means consuming less than 30 percent fat, and the American Heart Association concedes that this 30 percent guideline represents a compromise. At AHI we believe that a truly heart-wise diet includes no more than 20 percent fat. The food plan in the Diethrich Program, like the one which Dr. Ornish's patients followed, contains approximately 10 percent fat.

Such a plan is exceedingly strict. It includes virtually no meat, no fish, no egg yolks, no dairy products (except skim milk and nonfat yogurt), and no butter, margarine, oils, or mayonnaise. Instead, participants indulge in virtually limitless quantities of pasta, rice and other grains, beans, vegetables, and fruits in a wide variety of combinations and preparations. Hundreds of people on similar programs throughout the country affirm that eating this way allows for tasty, varied, interesting meals and that they successfully made the adjustment without feeling deprived. For the most part, however, heart disease had become a veritable executioner to these men and women and this food plan was literally their salvation. Because eating an ultralow-fat diet requires a radical change in habits, long-term success requires solid education and strong motivation.

Whether you should adopt such a strict program or begin on a more modest one is a decision you and your doctor will have to make based on your cholesterol level, health, and personality. In any

FAT AND CHOLESTEROL CONTENT
OF COMMON FOODS

FOOD	TOTAL FAT (GRAMS)	SATURATED FAT (GRAMS)	CHOLESTEROL (MILLIGRAMS)
Meat, Fish, Eggs			
(Unless otherwise noted, portion is 3 ounces, cooked weight, without added fat)			
Beef, flank steak	12.6	5.4	60
chuck roast	8.7	3.3	84
filet mignon	8.1	3.3	72
ground, extra lean	13.5	5.4	84
liver	4.2	1.5	330
Lamb, leg	5.7	3.6	75
rib	11.4	3.6	75
Bacon (1 ounce)	14.0	5.0	24
Canadian bacon (1 ounce)	2.4	0.8	16
Ham, extra lean	4.8	1.5	45
Pork tenderloin	4.2	1.5	78
Veal rib	5.4	1.8	108
Frankfurter, beef and pork (2 ounces)	16.6	6.2	28
chicken (2 ounces)	11.0	3.2	56
Chicken, breast, skinless	2.9	0.8	73
with skin	6.15	1.73	62
dark meat, skinless	7.5	2.1	75
Turkey, light meat, skinless	0.9	0.3	72
dark meat, skinless	3.6	1.2	96
Grouper	1.2	0.3	39
Salmon, fresh	6.3	1.2	42
Snapper	1.5	0.3	39
Tuna, white, canned in water	2.1	0.6	36
Lobster	0.6	trace	60
Shrimp	0.9	0.3	165
Egg, 1 whole, raw	5.6	1.7	213
Egg, 1 white, raw	trace	0	0

Dairy

Milk, skim (1 cup)	0.4	0.3	4
1% (1 cup)	2.6	1.6	10
Yogurt, nonfat	0.4	0.3	4
Ice milk (½ cup)	2.8	1.8	9
Half and half (1 tablespoon)	1.7	1.1	6
Sour cream (tablespoon)	2.5	1.6	5
Nondairy creamer (1 teaspoon)	0.7	0.7	0
Cheese, natural, (1 ounce) Brie, cheddar, Colby, Edam Gouda, Gruyère, Monterey, Parmesan, Roquefort, Swiss	9.4	6.0	30
Cheese, cottage, 1% (½ cup)	1.2	0.7	5

Fats and Oils

Butter (1 teaspoon)	4.1	2.5	11
Margarine, corn oil stick (1 teaspoon)	3.8	0.6	0
Diet (1 teaspoon)	1.9	0.3	0
Peanut butter (2 teaspoons)	5.5	0.9	0
Mixed nuts, dry roasted (3 tablespoons)	14.6	2.0	0

Breads and Grains

Bagel (3-inch diameter)	2.6	unknown	unknown
English muffin (½)	0.6	unknown	unknown
Bread, white (1 slice)	0.9	0.2	unknown
Corn flakes (1 ounce)	0.1	0	0
Shredded Wheat (1 large biscuit)	0.3	0	0
Oatmeal (1 cup)	2.4	0.4	0
Rice (1 cup)	0.2	0	0
Spaghetti (1 cup)	0.6		unknown

Vegetables and Fruits

Apple (2¾-inch diameter)	0.5	0.1	0
Banana	0.3	0	0
Cantaloupe (1 cup)	0.4	0	0
Mango (half)	0.3	0	0

Starchy vegetables (½ cup)			
potatoes, corn, lima beans,			
plantain, squash, yams	0		0
Other vegetables (½ to 1 cup)	0.2	0	0

Values are approximate.
Source: USDA Provisional Table on the Fatty Acids and Cholesterol Content of Selected Foods, 1984, as adapted from *The AHA Low Fat, Low Cholesterol Cookbook*.

case, if diet and exercise alone do not lower your cholesterol sufficiently within six months, the American Heart Association, the National Cholesterol Education Program, and most other experts recommend you consider taking cholesterol-lowering drugs. These drugs are prescribed in addition to a low-fat diet, never as a replacement.

As our knowledge about the correlation between diet and cholesterol levels has increased, we have learned that although lowering blood cholesterol is the goal, solely counting milligrams of dietary cholesterol will probably not achieve it. Since the saturated fat we consume affects the liver's ability to regulate blood levels of cholesterol even more than dietary cholesterol, and since all fats contain some proportion of saturated fat, the easiest way to lower blood cholesterol is by reducing total fat. As a rule of thumb, you should consume no more than 300 milligrams of cholesterol a day. But if you avoid foods that are especially high in cholesterol, such as organ meats and egg yolks (one egg yolk, for example, contains 213 milligrams of cholesterol), and limit your total fat intake sufficiently, you will automatically keep your cholesterol consumption down.

Once you and your doctor determine what percentage of total fat your diet should contain, you can set about achieving your goal. One gram of fat contains nine calories. Roughly speaking, therefore, a 10-percent-fat diet contains approximately one gram of fat for every one hundred calories you consume. Likewise, a 20-percent-fat diet contains about two grams of fat per one hundred calories, a 30-percent-fat diet contains about three grams of fat, and so on. If you typically eat 2,000 calories a day, forty grams of fat would give you a just less than 20-percent-fat diet, healthy by most standards.

With a precise idea of the fat content in various foods, you can balance your diet by offsetting a selection relatively high in fat with one that is much lower. To get a more precise calculation of the percent of fat you are consuming, follow this procedure:

1. Scan the food label to find the grams of total fat per serving and the number of calories per serving.
2. To calculate the number of calories from fat, multiply the number of grams of fat per serving by 9.
3. To calculate the percentage of calories from fat, divide the number of calories from fat by the total calories per serving.

Here's an example:

1. One tablespoon of Hellmann's cholesterol-free reduced-calorie mayonnaise contains 50 calories and 5 grams of fat.
2. Since there are 5 grams of fat and each gram contains 9 calories, there are 5 × 9 or 45 calories from fat.
3. 45 calories from fat divided by 50 calories per serving = 0.9 or 90 percent of calories from fat.

Raised in the American tradition, we can consume forty grams of fat, 20 percent of a 2,000-calorie diet, without even realizing it. For example, a salad with two tablespoons of a typical oil- or mayonnaise-based dressing contains thirty-six grams of fat, and we haven't even mentioned the margarine on your breakfast bagel. (Bagels themselves have virtually no fat, but one tablespoon of margarine contains 11 grams of fat.) But with a little knowledge and a few tricks, you can cut back substantially on the fat in your diet without feeling punished.

To achieve a 20- to 25-percent-fat diet, begin by cutting way back on visible fats: butter, margarine, cream cheese, oil, mayonnaise, salad dressing. Even if you use reduced-fat products, measure the fat you use in teaspoons rather than tablespoons (three teaspoons equals one tablespoon), and limit yourself to six units per day, each unit defined as follows: one teaspoon of margarine or oil; one and one-half teaspoons oil- or mayonnaise-based salad dressings; two teaspoons of reduced-fat mayonnaise. Try apple butter on your bagel in the morning instead of margarine. For sautéing, use a quick spritz of cooking oil spray, which now comes in butter flavor, olive oil, and corn oil varieties. Alternatively, put your favorite cooking oil into a bottle with a spray pump, and use this to lightly coat your pan. Choose a heavy pan and lower the flame to keep your food from burning. Steam your

HELLMANN'S® CHOLESTEROL FREE REDUCED CALORIE MAYONNAISE

CALORIES PER SERVING	
Hellmann's® Cholesterol Free............................	50
Regular Mayonnaise......................................	100

Enjoy great taste that is 100% cholesterol free, half the calories, and low in sodium. Use Hellmann's® Cholesterol Free on sandwiches and in all your favorite recipes.

NUTRITION INFORMATION PER SERVING

Serving size:	1 tablespoon (15 grams)
Servings per container (Pt.)	32
Calories	50
Protein	0 gram
Carbohydrate	1 gram
Fat	5 grams
Percent of calories from fat	92
Polyunsaturated	2 grams
Saturated	1 gram
Cholesterol	0 mg (0 mg/100 g)
Sodium	80 milligrams

Source: Courtesy Best Foods.

vegetables in a steamer or saucepan or microwave them. Store your canned chicken broth in the refrigerator to make the fat solidify and rise to the top, so you can skim it off easily. If you buy salad dressing, choose the nonfat varieties. If you make your own, combine vinegar and seasonings separately from the oil. Dress your salad with one teaspoon of oil per person and as much vinegar mixture as you like. If you find the dressing too strong, dilute the vinegar with a little water. If you prefer mayonnaise-based dressings, mix the mayonnaise with an equal part of nonfat yogurt or nonfat cottage cheese whirled smooth in the blender. As you peruse the new crop of low-fat cookbooks and low-fat cooking columns that now appear regularly in newspapers and magazines, you'll undoubtedly pick up other tricks.

In addition, limit your animal protein to six ounces a day. For good health, women and men need only 0.8–1.2 grams of protein for every kilogram they weigh. For a 110-pound woman, this translates into a daily allotment of three ounces of meat protein (including fish and chicken) plus two glasses of milk. (There are 7 grams of protein per ounce of meat or cup of milk.) You could get an equivalent amount of protein from five ounces of meat protein or four ounces of meat protein plus six servings of grain. By eating more protein than your body needs, you consume unnecessary fat because animal protein is inherently high in fat. Prepared without any additional fat, skin-free white meat turkey contains 17 percent fat; white meat chicken, also without skin, is 24 percent fat; a lean hamburger is 61 percent fat; whole-milk yogurt is 48 percent fat; an egg, whose fat comes entirely from the yolk, is 64 percent fat; Swiss cheese is 66 percent fat.

But you don't have to ban these foods from your diet. If you love red meat, choose the leanest cuts: eye of the round or flank steak, for example. Try the "select" grade, which has less fat than "choice" grade, and limit your portion to three ounces cooked weight, a piece about the size of a deck of playing cards. Choose fish or chicken more frequently, and, again, keep your portion to the same size: three ounces (half a moderate-size salmon steak or half a chicken breast). Because fish has omega-3 fatty acids, which lower triglycerides and help prevent clotting and coronary artery spasm, even the fattiest varieties such as salmon are thought to be healthful. Because they are high in omega-3 fatty acids but low in saturated fat and calories, shell-fish—including shrimp and lobster—are acceptable even though they are relatively high in cholesterol. Scallops and clams are lowest in fat, calories, and cholesterol. Chicken and turkey are also lower in fat than red meat, even when cooked with the skin. A 1985 study funded by the National Broiler Council and referenced in the *New England Journal of Medicine* documents that chicken cooked in its skin absorbs no fat from the skin. For succulent chicken, try browning it under the broiler using no added fat, then complete the cooking by baking at a lower temperature or transferring the chicken to the microwave. Remove the skin before eating. Since a three-ounce portion of protein is bound to look skimpy, especially at first, add a soup, salad, or additional vegetable to amplify the meal. With another course, a fuller plate, and additional variety, you're less likely to feel deprived. Alternatively, slice your protein thin, stir-fry it with a mixture of vegetables, and serve over rice or pasta.

In addition, go for low-fat or nonfat dairy products. Choose the nonfat versions of yogurt and cottage cheese. Explore the nonfat cheese substitutes; they're improving. And opt for skim milk, which is virtually fat free, rather than one percent milk, which contains approximately 23 percent fat calories.

As you reduce the amount of fat and protein you eat, you will need to increase your complex carbohydrates (beans, grains, and other starchy vegetables), other vegetables, and fruits. Keep on the lookout for interesting meatless entrees. Develop your repertoire of pasta, risotto, and vegetable main dishes that incorporate cheese or other animal protein as a condiment. Explore bulghur wheat, couscous, brown rice, kasha, navy beans, kidney beans, and black beans, lentils, chick-peas, black-eyed peas, and split peas. Use them for salads, soups, and stews. And have lots of leftovers around for snacking. As you eat less fat, you are likely to become hungry more frequently. But you will probably find that the less fat you consume, the more you can snack on carbohydrates without gaining weight. (This phenomenon is explained more fully in the weight loss section later in the chapter.)

Although nearly everyone could profit from a diet lower in fat, only 15 percent of the American population is doing anything about it, according to a 1991 survey by the National Cholesterol Education Program. And that number is down from 19 percent in 1986. The primary reason why people resist a low-fat diet is that it feels like punishment. Food is tremendously important to most of us. As infants, when hunger was our greatest pain, the satisfying milk and mother's soothing touch made a deep impression on our minds. From those earliest days, food has been synonymous with love and comfort. As adults, we use food to ease our anguish, reward our successes, salute our triumphs, and celebrate our joys. Food is central to every social, emotional, and cultural event. What's a movie without popcorn? A baseball game without a hot dog and beer? A romance without a candelight dinner for two?

You will be successful in modifying your diet only if you can do it without feeling deprived or punished. Accomplishing this feat relies on understanding how food satiates you emotionally as well as physically and revising your food choices to meet your emotional needs. Do you reach for the chips because you have the urge to munch? If so, try keeping your fridge supplied with a variety of raw vegetables that have been cleaned and cut and are ready for snacking. Do you go to the freezer to satisfy your sweet tooth? If so, keep your freezer stocked with nonfat yogurt, sorbet, fudgsicles, and frozen fruit juice bars.

Perhaps you enjoy cooking and salivate at the mere thought of creating a taste sensation. If so, go out of your way to select the freshest foods. Look for fish that has clear, bright eyes and shiny scales. Check the pull date on chicken packages and choose the one with the latest date; if you plan to freeze the chicken, wash it and repackage it first. Pick out the firmest, freshest fruits and vegetables. Discover the flavor burst of fresh herbs, which are readily available in supermarkets today; the richness of sauces made by reducing seasoned broth and wine; and the varied textures of unusual grains.

Do you worry that fat restriction will take all the fun out of cooking? Instead, take on the challenge. Spend some time perusing the growing selection of low-fat cookbooks (see Additional Resources) and learn the art of substitution: Use evaporated skim milk in recipes that call for cream and nonfat yogurt* in place of sour cream, replace gravies with stock and wine reductions thickened with a little cornstarch, use bulghur wheat instead of ground meat in chili. Set yourself the goal of trying one new recipe a week. Explore the Asian cuisines, which are inherently low in fat. Discover the unusual tastes of curry, cumin, and cardamom. If you approach a low-fat diet with a sense of adventure, you're likely to discover satisfying new dishes and appealing new tastes to replace the old favorites you're eating less frequently.

Perhaps your concern is for convenience. Happily, eating healthfully has never been easier. The retail market, ever eager to jump on a profitable bandwagon, has responded to demands for low-fat, low-sodium selections. In your supermarket freezer, refrigerator case, and open shelves you'll find a variety of prepared food under such labels as Healthy Choice and Le Menu Light Style. Check labels carefully and choose dishes made with less than three grams of fat for every one hundred calories.

Restaurants are responding as well. Many feature dishes made in compliance with American Heart Association guidelines; these are usually clearly marked on the menu. Restaurants that do not feature omelets made with egg substitutes or other special dishes are usually happy to answer questions about how food is prepared and to meet requests for steamed vegetables or broiled fish without butter. Even

* To keep yogurt from curdling, add 1 teaspoon cornstarch to each cup of nonfat yogurt in the following manner: Mix the cornstarch with one-fourth cup of yogurt. Add to remaining yogurt and mix thoroughly.

fast-food restaurants are heeding the call. New franchises featuring chicken barbecued without added fat and heart-healthy side dishes are burgeoning. In April 1991, McDonald's introduced the McLean Deluxe, a burger as low in fat as a Hardee's grilled chicken sandwich, which has 310 calories and about nine grams of fat. In addition, you can order salads and baked potatoes at Wendy's; baked fish and a baked potato at Long John Silver's; bagels at Dunkin Donuts; and nonfat yogurt at Dairy Queen. Fast-food restaurants willingly supply nutritional information about the foods they serve, too. McDonald's posts a chart in most shops. Burger King has brochures at the counter; they're free for the asking. Kentucky Fried Chicken will send you a brochure if you call 502-456-8300, ext. 8353, or write to KFC Corporation, Public Affairs Department, P.O. Box 32070, Louisville, KY 40232. Wendy's will answer nutritional questions if you call their customer service department at 1-800-443-7266.

As you peruse restaurant menus, avoid creations that are creamed, buttered, fried, breaded, scalloped, broasted, or prepared au gratin. Instead select dishes that are broiled, grilled, roasted, baked, steamed, or poached. Order sauces and dressings on the side, so you can control how much you consume.

And beware. Even chicken without the skin and fish can be laden with hidden fats. As a result, half a dozen chicken nuggets can have more fat than a hamburger. A fast-food fried chicken sandwich can contain as much fat as a pint and a half of ice cream.

In general, be leery of the word "light" and its various spellings. The FDA has not defined "light," which commonly refers to color and weight, and not necessarily to calorie or fat content. "Free" is another deceptive word. Since the FDA's definition of "free" is not synonymous with zero, foods called fat free may include small amounts of oil, eggs, or milk products. Check the label before you indulge indiscriminately.

As these illustrations reveal, advertisers have adopted some misleading practices to lure the health-conscious consumer. When cholesterol was first named as a villain, commercial bakers substituted coconut and palm oils for butter and touted their cakes and cookies as cholesterol-free. However, these vegetable oils are highly saturated and can raise blood cholesterol levels even more than animal fat. In the next shift of strategy, commercial bakers boasted "no tropical oils," as they switched to soybean, corn, and safflower oils that had been hydrogenated. However, hydrogenation, which produces a crisper product, makes unsaturated oils behave as though they were saturated, both in the cookie and in the bloodstream.

In another pitch to the health-conscious consumer, advertisers claim foods to be nearly free of fat based on weight rather than the more legitimate proportion of total calories. To understand the difference, think about the implications of mixing a tablespoon of oil into a glass of water. By weight, the proportion of oil is small. But in nutritional terms, 100 percent of calories come from fat. Similarly, whole milk contains 4 percent fat by weight and could therefore claim to be 96 percent fat free. However, whole milk contains eight grams of fat, or 48 percent of its 150 calories from fat—not such a healthy choice.

If you want to succeed in changing your diet forever, approach the challenge with a sense of moderation. We cannot emphasize moderation strongly enough. Countless people have tackled change with zeal only to fail in the end. They have spent hours reading labels in the grocery store, denied themselves all their favorite foods, avoided social occasions because they were afraid to spring a dietary trap, and felt guilty if they cheated. More than anything else, they made themselves miserable. Before long, they abandoned their resolve and returned to their bad habits. You are much more likely to be successful if you adapt gradually. If you have a passion for red meat, permit yourself to enjoy it once or twice a week. If you've never had a vegetarian dinner, ease meatless meals into your repetoire gradually. And every once in a while, splurge on your favorite dessert. The idea is not to mourn the permanent loss of chocolate cake but to discover enough delicious, healthy foods that you will miss it less and less.

Increasing Fiber

In the mid-seventies, diabetes researcher James W. Anderson, M.D., and his colleagues at the University of Kentucky discovered that a diet high in carbohydrates and plant fiber but low in fat regulated blood sugar levels by slowing the absorption of carbohydrates. As a result, patients with Type I (juvenile) diabetes could reduce their daily insulin dosage; most Type II diabetics who needed insulin were able to stop taking the drug after just three weeks on the diet, and by following the diet many remained insulin independent for twelve years or more. Serendipitously, the researchers discovered that their patients' cholesterol levels dropped as much as 30 percent, and a new concept in cholesterol management was born.

DIETARY FIBER

FOOD	DIETARY FIBER (GRAMS)	FOOD	DIETARY FIBER (GRAMS)
Cereals		beans, lima, cooked	
All Bran (½ cup)	13.2	(½ cup)	3.1
Bran Buds	12.0	beans, pinto, canned	
40% Bran Flakes (½ cup)	2.6	(½ cup)	5.7
brown rice, cooked		broccoli ½ cup	3.3
(½ cup)	1.7	cabbage, cooked (½ cup)	2.6
corn bran (½ cup)	4.0	carrots (½ cup)	1.8
corn flakes (½ cup)	1.4	cauliflower (½ cup)	0.8
Fiber One (½ cup)	18.0	celery (½ cup)	1.1
Grapenuts (½ cup)	4.4	corn, boiled (1 ear)	3.1
Miller's unprocessed bran		cucumber (1 medium)	1.5
(1 ounce)	4.6	lettuce, iceberg (½ cup)	0.4
(sprinkle on food or		peas, cooked (½ cup)	8.3
mix with juice)		potatoes, raw, boiled	
Nutrigrain Wheat (½ cup)	1.4	(1 medium)	3.0
oat bran, cooked (½ cup)	2.1	spinach (½ cup)	1.0
oatmeal, cooked (½ cup)	1.8	tomato (1 small)	1.0
Rice Krispies (½ cup)	0.6		
Shredded Wheat, 1 biscuit	3.4	**Fruits**	
Special K (½ cup)	0.4	apple, delicious (1 small)	3.4
Wheaties (½ cup)	1.3	apricots (2 medium)	1.8
Wheat Chex (½ cup)	1.7	banana (1 small)	2.0
		cantaloupe (¼ small)	0.9
Breads (1 slice)		cherries (15 large)	1.1
pumpernickel	0.6	grapes (10 medium)	0.5
rye (no seeds)	0.4	orange, navel (1 small)	2.2
Rye Krisp crackers (2)	1.5	pear, Bosc (1 medium)	4.8
white bread	0.2	plums (10 small)	2.1
whole wheat bread	1.3	raspberries (½ cup)	1.9
		strawberries (½ cup)	1.7
Vegetables (raw, except as noted)		blueberries (½ cup)	2.5
beans, green, canned		prunes (5 small)	4.4
(½ cup)	1.8		
beans, kidney, canned			
(½ cup)	5.8		

Source: *Dietary Fiber: The Experts' View, Intestinal Disorders.* Sponsored by Tufts University School of Nutrition and published by KPR Infor/Media Corp., 1987. Chart by Chesley Hines, Jr., M.D., Clinical Associate Professor, Tulane University School of Medicine and Louisiana State Medical Center.

Subsequent research showed that a diet very high in oat bran and other water-soluble fibers—unrealistically high in the context of American eating habits, Dr. Anderson admitted—can lower LDL cholesterol by 58 percent and raise HDL cholesterol 82 percent. Other studies reveal that generous consumption of oat bran and legumes—peas and beans—can lower total cholesterol 20 percent, lower LDL 25 percent, and raise HDL 15 percent. Taking one teaspoonful of psyllium hydrophilic mucilloid (found in Metamucil and similar products) three times a day can yield similar results, although doing it with diet is preferable.

The fiber that controls cholesterol is *soluble*, as opposed to *insoluble*, and is found in rice bran, rolled oats, carrots, fruit pectin, barley, and legumes, in addition to oat bran and psyllium. Consequently, a heart-smart diet includes generous proportions of whole-grain cereals, brown rice, fruit with peel, and varieties of beans (pinto, navy, kidney) and other legumes (such as black-eyed peas, split peas, lentils).

Every healthy diet also includes substantial insoluble fiber, found largely in vegetables, unrefined wheat, and most grains. This kind of fiber speeds foods through the intestinal tract, increases fecal bulk, and delays digestion and absorption of carbohydrates. Insoluble fiber therefore helps control constipation, decreases the likelihood of serious intestinal disorders, and reduces the risk of colon cancer.

Despite the implications of TV ads to the contrary, you will not cure high cholesterol with a bowl of oatmeal in the morning. In fact, you probably cannot consume enough fiber on a regular basis to achieve the results Dr. Anderson saw in his studies. Nevertheless, a diet high in soluble and insoluble fiber can only help your health. While Americans typically get 10 to 20 grams of fiber in their daily diet, the National Cancer Institute recommends 20 to 30 grams per day. The Dietary Guidelines for Americans, issued by the U.S. Department of Agriculture and the Department of Health and Human Services, recommends that we achieve this goal by following this food plan:

- vegetables: three to five servings, one serving defined as 1 cup of raw leafy greens or ½ cup of other selections
- fruits: two to four servings, one serving defined as one medium apple, orange or banana; ½ cup berries or cut-up fruit; six ounces juice

- whole grains: six to eleven servings, one serving defined as one slice of bread; ½ roll, bagel, or English muffin; 1 ounce of dry cereal; ½ cup rice or other grain, pasta, or cooked cereal

Limiting Salt

When we eat salt, or, more precisely, sodium chloride, our bodies retain water. For people with heart failure or kidney disease, this is a serious problem, because retaining water increases the volume of fluid in the blood vessels and, in turn, increases the strain on the already compromised heart and kidneys. (See Chapter 7 for more on heart failure.) Water retention can also contribute to filling the lungs with fluid.

Although we once thought that the increased volume of fluid in the blood vessels would harm anyone with high blood pressure, we now know better. Eating salt—that is, sodium—does not cause high blood pressure and it aggravates the condition only in perhaps half of all hypertensive people, those who are sensitive to salt. When people with sodium-sensitive hypertension cut back substantially on their salt intake—that is, when they avoid pickles, chips, fast food, and other salty foods and when they add no salt while cooking or at the table—they can lower their blood pressure by about 5 millimeters of mercury. Over time, the benefits of this small reduction are substantial.

If you have high blood pressure, try reducing the sodium in your diet for several weeks—it will take this long to see some results—and see if your blood pressure responds. If it does, then restricting your salt intake is beneficial. If your blood pressure stays the same, your kidneys are excreting the excess salt from your body normally, and restricting your salt is unnecessary; your high blood pressure needs to be controlled in another way.

General wisdom suggests that, for everyone, less salt is better than more. Americans commonly consume 8,000 to 12,000 milligrams of sodium a day. (One teaspoon of salt contains 2,300 milligrams of sodium.) For good health, the body requires only 1,100 to 3,300 milligrams. People who have no health requirement for limiting their sodium would be wise to hold their intake to 3,000 to 4,000 milligrams a day. Certainly, if you ever have to restrict your salt, being accustomed to eating less salt will make the transition less punitive. Although salt is a flavor enhancer, it is a learned taste, and millions of people will attest to the truth that it can be unlearned. Adjusting your taste buds will take about three months.

If you must restrict your salt, ask your physician or a registered dietitian whether it is safe for you to use light salt, one-third to one-half of which (depending on brand) is composed of potassium chloride, or salt substitutes. Begin eliminating salt by avoiding olives, chips, and other highly salted foods (most of which are high in fat as well). Some people must hold their salt intake to three grams a day, the amount sanctioned by the American Heart Association. To accomplish this goal, you probably do not need to buy foods that are specifically low in sodium, but you should limit the salt you add while cooking and avoid using the salt shaker at the table. If you have serious heart failure and must reduce your salt even more, you will need to restrict yourself to low-sodium foods, including soups, tomato sauce, and other canned goods, and avoid the salt shaker completely.

To keep from feeling punished and deprived, approach salt reduction with the same sense of moderation and exploration as fat reduction. Some people find that when they cook with salt substitutes, their food takes on a bitter, metallic taste. If you add salt substitutes at the table instead of at the stove, you're more likely to find it palatable. But if salt substitutes don't appeal to you, reach instead for the pepper mill, Lawry's Salt-Free, Mrs. Dash's seasoning mix, or another salt alternative. Experiment with several and see how they strike you. Try recipes from a low-salt cookbook.

Next, unless your doctor insists that you go off sodium cold turkey, decrease the salt in your cooking gradually. If you are on a 3,000 milligram program, aim to add no more than one-half teaspoon of salt (1,150 milligrams sodium) to your food per day. All the while, add more ample quantities of herbs and spices. Experiment with fresh herbs. And when you open a new jar of dried herbs, instead of storing it in the pantry, keep it in the freezer, where it will retain its zing forever. In addition, you will reduce your salt intake if you use fresh or frozen vegetables (although some frozen vegetables have added salt—check labels) rather than canned varieties; make your own pasta sauces, soups, and pancake mixes; reduce your consumption of prepared foods; and rinse canned tuna and other canned foods with fresh water before using. If you choose the freshest possible fish, fruits, and vegetables, they will be flavorful on their own.

SODIUM CONTENT OF COMMON FOODS

FOOD	SODIUM (MILLIGRAMS)
Meat and Fish	
(3 ounces cooked weight, no salt added)	
Ground beef, extra lean	69
Ham, extra lean	1,023
Chicken, breast, skinless	59
Alaska King Crab	912
Flounder	90
Dairy	
Milk, skim (1 cup)	126
Yogurt, nonfat (1 cup)	174
Cheese, American (1 ounce)	406
Cheese, natural (1 ounce)	
blue, Brie, cheddar, Colby, Edam, Gouda, Gruyère,	
Monterey, Parmesan, Roquefort, Swiss	176
Grains	
Bagel (3-inch diameter)	360
40% Bran Flakes (1 ounce)	264
Shredded Wheat (1 large biscuit)	0
Oatmeal, cooked without salt (1 cup)	1
Rice, cooked without salt (1 cup)	4
Fruits and Vegetables	2–63
Fresh vegetables (½ cup, cooked)	
Canned vegetables (unless specifically prepared	
without salt)	High
Cantaloupe (1 cup)	14
Honeydew (1 cup)	17
Other fresh fruits	0–6
Fats and Oils	
Corn oil margarine (1 teaspoon)	44
Diet margarine (1 teaspoon)	46

Mayonnaise (1 tablespoon)	78
French dressing (1 tablespoon)	214

Prepared Soups

Chicken noodle soup, canned (1 cup)	1,107
Minestrone, canned (1 cup, prepared with water)	911
Tomato rice soup, canned (1 cup, prepared with water)	815

Fast Food

Hot dog (1)	636
Cheeseburger (1 regular)	672
Tuna sub	1,288
Hot fudge sundae	177

Values are approximate.

Source: USDA *Nutritive Value of American Foods in Common Units*, Agricultural Handbook No. 456, 1975, and USDA Provisional Table on the Nutrient Content of Fast Foods, 1984, as adapted from *The AHA Low Fat, Low Cholesterol Cookbook*.

Getting Enough Calcium

Twenty-five million Americans, 80 percent of them women and most of them white, have osteoporosis, a condition in which bones become thin, porous, and fragile. A silent disease, osteoporosis ravages the bones painlessly until they crumble. As their spines gradually collapse and bend into a "dowager's hump," some women with osteoporosis develop a characteristic hunched-over look. Others first discover they have the condition when they break a bone. They may suffer spontaneous fractures of the spine, which are excruciating and untreatable. Or they may fall and fracture a hip, which often requires surgery and may cause permanent disability.

Bone cells are in a continuous state of degeneration and regeneration. When we are young, bones build up more rapidly than they break down. We build our greatest amount of bone mass during the teenage years. Except in women who are estrogen deficient, bones continue to increase in mass, albeit more slowly, during the twenties and thirties. Once women lose estrogen at menopause, their bones begin to disintegrate more quickly than they regenerate, and overall bone mass diminishes.

A calcium-rich diet helps to prevent the bone loss that can lead to osteoporosis. Research also suggests that calcium helps to control high blood pressure, and an Argentinian study published late in 1991 found that women who took 2,000 milligrams of supplemental calcium daily were able to prevent high blood pressure during their pregnancies, a serious hazard for mother and baby. A word of caution: 2,000 milligrams of calcium is approximately double the recommended intake during pregnancy and can set the stage for kidney stones. If you are pregnant, do not take supplemental calcium or any other medication without consulting your doctor.

To protect against osteoporosis, menstruating women and postmenopausal women taking estrogen need 1,000 milligrams of calcium a day. Postmenopausal women taking less than 0.625 milligrams of Premarin or its equivalent need 1,500 milligrams daily. Although skim milk contains 300 milligrams of calcium per cup and low-fat plain yogurt contains 415 milligrams per cup, it is difficult to consume sufficient calcium when you're trying to cut down on high-fat, high-cholesterol dairy products. Some vegetables, notably broccoli and collard greens, are rich in calcium. Since vitamin D increases absorption, consuming milk products that are fortified with vitamin D will help you get the most out of the calcium you take in.

If you don't get enough calcium in your diet, you should take 500, 1,000, or 1,500 milligrams of calcium supplements daily, depending on your individual needs. Calcium tablets come in three common forms: calcium carbonate, calcium lactate, and calcium citrate. Ask your doctor or registered dietitian which is best for you. Be aware that some supplements, notably dolomite, contain lead. Whichever compound is recommended, the tablet you buy should dissolve in water within thirty minutes or your body may not be able to make use of it. Although most preparations don't need to be dissolved before you take them, you should test a tablet when you buy a new brand. Since vitamin D increases calcium absorption, choosing a tablet enriched with vitamin D is a good idea. Take 500 milligrams of calcium at a time, preferably after a meal.

Interestingly, women raised on a traditional Chinese diet suffer surprisingly little osteoporosis. Apparently, animal protein, fat, and phosphates (prevalent in meats and carbonated beverages) interfere with the body's ability to utilize calcium. Vegetarians excrete less calcium in their urine than people who eat animal protein.

CALCIUM CONTENT OF CALCIUM-RICH FOODS*

FOOD	CALCIUM (MILLIGRAMS)
Dairy Products	
Milk (Unless otherwise noted, portion is 1 cup.)	
Buttermilk, cultured	285
1% lowfat	300
Skim	302
Skim milk powder (¼ cup)	377
Cheese (Unless otherwise noted, portion is 1 oz.)	
American, pasteurized process	124
Blue	150
Brick	191
Cheddar	204
Colby	194
Cottage, 1% lowfat (½ cup)	69
Gouda	198
Mozzarella, part skim	183
Muenster	203
Parmesan, grated (1 tbsp.)	69
Ricotta, part skim, ½ cup	337
Swiss	272
Yogurt (1 cup)	
Skim with nonfat dry milk solids, plain	452
Lowfat with nonfat dry milk solids, plain	415
Lowfat with nonfat dry milk solids, fruit	314
Frozen desserts (½ cup)	
Ice milk, vanilla	88
Ice milk, vanilla soft serve	137
Sherbet, orange	57
Nondairy Products or Foods	
Oysters, cooked by moist heat (3 oz.)	76
Salmon, Sockeye, canned with bones (3 oz.)	203
Sardines, canned in tomato sauce with bones (1 large)	91
Tofu, raw, firm (½ cup)	258

Grains

Cornbread, from mix (1 piece)	133
Pancakes, 4″ diameter (3 extra light)	133
Fortified dry cereal (1 cup)	up to 98 (depending on brand)

Vegetables

Beans, black turtle, boiled (1 cup)	103
Beans, baked, vegetarian, canned (1 cup)	128
Beans, great northern, boiled (1 cup)	121
Beans, red kidney, canned (1 cup)	62
Broccoli, boiled (½ cup)	89
Cabbage, chinese, shredded (½ cup)	79
Collard greens, from raw (½ cup)	179
Kale, from frozen (½ cup)	90
Turnip greens, boiled (½ cup)	125

* Dairy products are the best sources of calcium, but many are high in fat.
  Source: Jean A. T. Pennington, *Food Values of Portions Commonly Used*, 15th edition (New York: Harper & Row, 1989).

Getting Enough Iron

After menopause, women need ten milligrams of iron a day. Menstruating women need fifteen milligrams, and an estimated 10 percent of menstruating women don't get enough iron. Moreover, anemia is a common problem after heart surgery. Since iron is most abundant in and absorbable from red meat and other foods high in fat and cholesterol, you may need to make a special effort to get enough of this element as you adopt a low-fat diet.

Some enriched cereals provide 100 percent of the daily required allowance. Choose cereals, breads, pastas, and grains that are fortified with iron. Whole-grain cereal, dark green leafy vegetables (kale, collard greens, mustard greens), dried beans and peas, and dried fruits are also good low-fat sources. Although iron from vegetables is not absorbed as efficiently as iron from meat, eating small amounts of veal or fish with black beans can almost double the iron absorbed from the vegetables. Since vitamin C also enhances iron absorption, eating tomatoes, citrus fruits, and other foods high in vitamin C in the same meal as iron-rich foods will help you utilize the iron you consume. In addition, if you cook your food slowly in cast-iron pots, some of the iron from the pot will be imparted to the food, especially acid-rich foods such as tomatoes. Leave the skin on vegetables and fruits while they cook, use small amounts of water in cooking, avoid soaking vegetables for any length of time, and whenever possible, save that water and add it to soups and stews.

Even if your diet is high in iron, if you are anemic, you may need to take a multivitamin or iron supplements. Your physician will probably prescribe ferrous sulfate and recommend that you take it with a glass of orange juice or 250 milligrams of vitamin C. Iron tablets can cause black bowel movements, constipation, and gas. To avoid constipation, be sure your diet is rich in fiber. If you have problems, consult your physician.

Limiting Caffeine and Avoiding Other Stimulants

Caffeine, which is found in coffee, tea, colas, cocoa, chocolate, and some medications, has been associated with increased cholesterol, irregular heartbeat, and increased incidence of heart attacks. However, the latest data, including separate studies conducted in Toronto and at Brigham and Women's Hospital in Boston suggest that these associations might not be valid. Although caffeine temporarily raises blood pressure and increases heart rate, coffee does not cause high blood pressure, probably because regular users develop a tolerance. Coffee has also been blamed for raising cholesterol, but the culprit here appears to the method of preparation. When coffee is dripped through a filter, rather than boiled, it does not appear to affect cholesterol.

At AHI, we have found that eliminating coffee can be strikingly effective in controlling arrhythmias, especially in women. But in a small study of patients hospitalized with arrhythmias, coffee did not trigger any problems. As to whether it contributes to causing heart attacks, the evidence is evenly mixed. In 1986, one large observational study, combined research by Johns Hopkins University and the National Center for Health Statistics, showed that the more coffee the participants drank, the more likely they were to be stricken. But 1990 results of the Harvard School of Public Health Survey, involving nearly 46,000 people, exonerated the brew.

If there was any connection between coffee and heart attacks, this study suggests, the villain was *decaffeinated* coffee, which was correlated

IRON CONTENT OF SELECTED FOODS

FOOD	IRON (MILLIGRAMS)
Meat, Poultry, and Fish, Cooked	
Clams (3 ounces)	23.8
Liver, pork (3 ounces)	15.2
Liver, chicken (3 ounces)	7.2
Mussels (3 ounces)	5.7
Oysters, canned (3 ounces)	5.7
Sardines, canned (3 ounces)	5.6
Liver, beef (3 ounces)	5.3
Tuna (3 ounces)	2.7
Shrimp (3 ounces)	2.6
Beef, round steak (3 ounces)	2.5
Trout (3 ounces)	2.0
Tofu, fried (3 ounces)	1.9
Chicken, dark (3 ounces)	1.1
Chicken, light (3 ounces)	0.9
Egg, whole (1 large)	0.7
Fruits	
Apricots, dried (¼ cup)	1.5
Raisins (¼ cup)	0.8
Watermelon (3 cups)	0.8
Strawberries (1 cup)	0.6
Vegetables	
Beans, navy (½ cup)	2.6
Beans, white (½ cup)	2.5
Spinach, canned (½ cup)	2.5
Beans, kidney (½ cup)	2.3
Beans, baby lima (½ cup)	2.0
Asparagus spears, cooked (1 cup)	1.8
Green peas, canned (½ cup)	1.8
Spinach, raw (1 cup)	1.5
Lettuce (¼ medium head)	0.7
Cauliflower, raw (1 cup)	0.6
Mustard greens, cooked (½ cup)	0.5

Bread and Cereal Products

Cereal, ready-to-eat and cooked	(level of iron varies with fortification or enrichment)
Bread and rolls	(level of iron varies with fortification or enrichment)

Miscellaneous

Blackstrap molasses (1 tablespoon)	3.2
Popcorn, popped (3 cups)	0.6

Source: U.S. Department of Health and Human Services.

GOOD SOURCES OF VITAMIN C*

Oranges or orange juice	Asparagus
Grapefruit or grapefruit juice	Bell peppers, green and red
Melons	Broccoli
Strawberries	Brussels sprouts
Pineapple or enriched juice	Cabbage
Enriched apple juice	Cauliflower
Lemons	Dark green vegetables: kale, collards,
Tomatoes	watercress, turnip greens, spinach, chard

* Since vitamin C enhances the absorption of iron, it's a good idea to eat one or more of these foods in the same meal as foods rich in iron.
Source: Arizona Heart Institute.

with some increased risk for heart attack and stroke. A Stanford study also pointed a finger at decaffeinated coffee when it showed that those who drank more than three cups a day had higher levels of LDL cholesterol. Clearly, the jury is still out. Unless your doctor recommends otherwise, you can probably drink two cups of coffee or other caffeinated drinks per day without danger.

If you need to avoid caffeine, be aware that it lurks in some odd places. Some aspirin compounds (including the original formulas for Empirin, Excedrin, and Anacin), and some cold medications contain caffeine. Before taking any over-the-counter medication, check the label.

Although you may be able to tolerate caffeine, there is no room in any healthy life-style for stronger stimulants, including nicotine (we'll talk more about smoking later in this chapter), cocaine, and amphetamines. They increase your risk of heart disease, exacerbate irregular heart rhythms, and trigger the fight-or-flight response.

Limiting Alcohol

Like the evidence on caffeine, the evidence on alcohol is mixed and controversial. Studies have indicted alcohol's potential to raise blood pressure, to cause strokes resulting from ruptured blood vessels in the brain, and to harm the heart muscle. Apart from heart disease, alcohol has been correlated to increased incidence of breast cancer and damage to the nervous system, liver, and pancreas. Alcohol is also fattening: 100 percent empty calories.

But studies have shown that moderate consumption of alcohol can raise HDL cholesterol. While some of this research reveals that the component of HDL that alcohol raises is not the same component associated with heart disease risk, this finding is not consistent. In the Nurses Health Study of 87,000 women, those who indulged in 3 to 9 drinks a week had half as much coronary heart disease as those who did not drink, a correlation the researchers called "remarkable." These researchers theorize that in addition to raising HDL, alcohol may influence blood clotting in a number of ways. It may help slow the ability of blood platelets to clot, interact with aspirin to enhance its effects, stimulate the release of natural clot-buster tPA, and lower the level of fibrinogen, a component of the blood that stimulates clotting. There is also some evidence that modest drinking reduces the risk of strokes caused by blockages in the arteries leading to the brain.

Some physicians feel that a glass of wine at night is therapeutic. Others feel that, especially for patients with heart failure, alcohol is poison. Unless you are overweight, have elevated blood sugar, or high triglycerides, one drink a day (12 ounces of light beer, 4 ounces of wine, or 1½ ounces of hard liquor) is probably safe, but check with your doctor to be sure.

EXERCISING REGULARLY

With all the talk about exercise and cardiovascular fitness, it's hard to believe that, not many years ago, exercise was thought to be bad for the heart. Contrary to practices today, where patients are up and walking within a couple of days after a heart attack, as recently as the 1950s, heart attack patients routinely spent 6 to 8 weeks in bed. Thinking began to change after a British researcher discovered that the ticket takers on the London buses had much lower rates of heart disease than the drivers. Why? The ticket takers spent their days running up and down the stairs of London's double-decker red buses.

The findings have been confirmed over and over. Regular aerobic exercise helps the heart beat more efficiently. It also raises HDL cholesterol and lowers blood pressure. In addition, exercise helps prevent osteoporosis, has been associated with a decrease in cancer, and improves the body's metabolism of sugar, thereby decreasing the probability of diabetes. By burning calories, raising the metabolism, and reducing hunger, exercise can also help you lose weight. By moderating the craving for nicotine, it also helps you stop smoking and helps clear the lungs and bronchial tubes of toxic effects of passive smoke. And it helps prevent depression and fosters inner peace by purging the mind of stress and raising levels of endorphins, body chemicals that dull pain and elevate mood.

In 1988 a ten-year University of North Carolina study of three thousand women showed that those in poor shape were three times more likely to die of heart disease at an early age than those who were fit. An eight-year study by Steven Blair and his associates, published in the *Journal of the American Medical Association* in 1989, showed that physical fitness delayed disability and death from several chronic diseases. Among the 13,000 participants—men and women—those who exercised lived longer, more vigorous lives than those who did not. Still another project, published in *Circulation* in February 1991, demonstrated that regular physical activity lowers blood pressure in women up to age eighty-nine.

However, most women over the age of forty do not exercise. Only one-fifth of the adult population exercises sufficiently for cardiovascular fitness. And, according to the Framingham research, 66 percent of women over the age of seventy-five could not lift an object weighing more than ten pounds.

As people age, their muscles tend to grow weaker. Their hearts become less efficient, and their muscles receive less oxygen. The net result is loss of strength and endurance, which threatens the independence of many otherwise healthy people in their late sixties and seventies. Exercise can slow this decline and recapture lost vigor. Athletic people in their seventies can achieve the strength of people twenty to twenty-five years their junior. In addition, older people who are fit seem to recover from illness and surgery more quickly than those who have no physical reserve. As Dr. William Evans of Tufts University's USDA Human Nutrition Research Center on Aging observed, "There is no single group that can benefit from exercise more than the elderly."

Even people with heart failure can benefit from exercise. An Oxford University study showed that riding a stationary bicycle helped people with severe, chronic heart failure increase their strength and endurance. Their newfound stamina kept them from feeling short of breath and enabled them to accomplish more during the day.

Weight-bearing exercise is particularly important for preventing osteoporosis. It stimulates blood circulation through the bones, supplying the bone-building cells with ample nourishment. And it sparks microscopic electrical charges within the bone that stimulate the bone-building cells.

A fourteen-year study of six thousand University of Pennsylvania graduates also suggests that exercise plays an important part in preventing Type II diabetes. This research, conducted exclusively on men, unfortunately, and apparently the only study of its kind, showed that six hours of vigorous exercise a week or a comparable energy output through more moderate activity cut risk of developing diabetes in half. Exactly how these data extrapolate to women is difficult to say, but considering that women are more vulnerable to diabetes than men, this study further builds the case for exercise.

For cardiovascular fitness, *moderate* aerobic activity appears to prolong life and well-being best. Walking thirty minutes a day or sixty minutes three times a week at 3 to 3.5 miles an hour is sufficient to improve cardiac conditioning and raise your HDL levels. Alternatively, you could bike, roller-skate, jog, go cross-country skiing, take Jazzercise or aerobics classes, or swim. Because of their buoyancy in water, people who swim suffer fewer injuries; this exercise may be the best choice for people with bad backs, arthritis, and other disabilities. Water aerobics classes, which feature muscle toning as well as aerobic exercise, have become increasingly popular.

Whatever exercise you choose, plan to keep at it for twenty to sixty minutes three to five times a week. For a fit heart and lungs, the American College of Sports Medicine recommends that healthy adults exercise strenuously enough to raise their heart rate, as measured in beats per minute, to 60 to 90 percent of maximum. You can approximate your maximum heart rate by subtracting your age from 220. Before beginning, talk to your doctor about an exercise prescription appropriate for your age and health. Find out how high your pulse should beat at its peak of your activity and how long you should sustain that rate.

Before you begin your routine, take your pulse to establish a resting heart rate (Figure 10-1). Take it again two or three times during your routine to make sure you're exercising at the correct intensity. Then take it once again when you're finished to make sure you've cooled down sufficiently. Use your second and third finger to take your pulse, since your thumb has a strong pulse of its own and can confuse your count. Find the carotid pulse just below the crook of your neck or the radial pulse on the inside of your wrist just below the thumb joint. Using a clock or watch with a second counter, count your pulse (beginning with zero) for ten seconds and multiply by six. If you don't remember your six times table, you can count your pulse for six seconds and add a zero; however a six-second count is probably less accurate than a ten-second count. Alternatively, you can purchase a mechanical pulse meter. These devices, which vary in design, accuracy, and price, are sold in sporting goods stores beginning at about $70.

Before you begin each exercise session, spend three to five minutes stretching to limber up your body and prevent injuries. Begin any aerobics activity slowly, and gradually build the intensity until you reach your peak heart rate. Sustain your peak according to your physician's prescription and then gradually slow down. Finally, spend another three to five minutes stretching to cool down. Stretching after exercise when your muscles are warm will increase your flexibility, help keep your muscles from cramping later, and help your pulse slow gradually to your resting heart rate. If, at any time during exercise, you feel chest pain, shortness of breath, lightheadedness, or any other cardiac symptoms, stop immediately and call your doctor.

In recent years, studies have shown that, in addition to aerobic exercise, weight training is tremendously beneficial for young and old alike. For young women, there is increasing evidence that pumping iron is as essential for preventing osteoporosis as aerobic exercise. One forty-one-year-old woman, whose bone scan showed she had the thin, brittle bones of a seventy-year-old, increased her bone mass 2.5 percent in ten months, enough to provide some protection against fractures. For older people, lifting weights has a valuable pay-

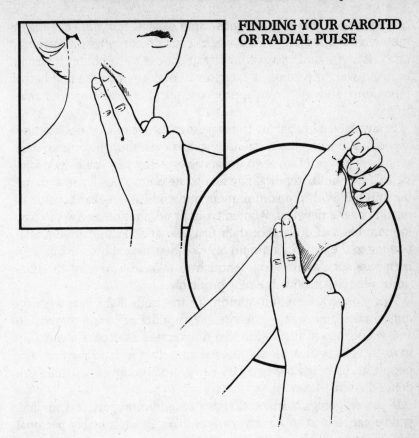

FINDING YOUR CAROTID OR RADIAL PULSE

FIGURE 10-1.

off in helping build strength and balance. One study showed that in less than eight weeks, a group of octogenarians had more than doubled their muscle strength by weight training. They walked faster, had better balance, and regained the capacity to climb stairs. This kind of improved strength and balance will help prevent falls and help you stay independent. Weight training will tone and define your muscles, but it won't make you bulk up as it does men.

If you don't do it carefully, however, weight training can cause serious injury. If you are healthy and belong to a fitness club, work with a knowledgeable exercise physiologist to establish a routine that is safe and beneficial. If you are ill or infirm, be sure to talk to your doctor first and work with a physical therapist. The American College of Sports Medicine recommends using weights to work each major muscle group at least twice a week. Your doctor, physical therapist, or exercise physiologist will help you choose the amount of weight to begin with, the kinds of exercises to perform, and the number of repetitions, and will set an appropriate plan for increasing your challenges.

In any exercise program, the biggest challenge of all is not quitting. Some health club chains stay in business even though some of their members pay as little as two dollars a year. How? By using the promise of a two-dollar renewal rate as a come-on to a costly initial membership fee. With the commitment and enthusiasm characteristic of turning over a new leaf, women typically commit themselves to paying hundreds of dollars for their first year at a health club. But after coming to the club for a month or two, they invariably drop out. Few members stick around long enough to take advantage of the two-dollar renewal, making the ploy profitable.

This gimmick is mute testimony to the truth that sweat is an acquired taste and regular exercise the product of strong motivation and willpower, at least at first. Even dedicated exercisers sometimes have to fight against inertia to get themselves up and moving. For people accustomed to sedentary living, no amount of scientific evidence can make exercise palatable.

If you're going to make exercise an enduring part of your life, you've got to find an activity that you like. This is a highly personal issue. Do you like to walk? Try walking early in the morning, late in the afternoon, or after dinner, and see which time seems to fit your schedule and your biorhythms best. Walk at the local mall when the weather is bad. Pick a different outside route each day to keep from getting bored. Walk with a friend before breakfast and stop at a café for a bagel before you go home. Walk after dinner and stop for frozen yogurt. Or walk alone and use the time for reflection and introspection. One way or another, make exercise a priority and schedule it into your agenda.

If you don't like walking, try indoor cross-country skiing machines, stationary bikes, rowing machines, low-impact aerobics, step aerobics, stair-climbing machines, or water aerobics. Exercise classes for older people, the overweight, and other special groups are sprouting; see what's available in your area. If you like aerobics classes but find the music too loud, try ear plugs. If you find exercise machines boring, watch television or listen to the radio while you work out. Alternatively, borrow an absorbing book on tape from the library and permit yourself to listen only while you're exercising.

In addition to being enjoyable, a successful exercise program must be convenient. If it's hard to set time aside for exercise, work it into your busy day. Instead of taking the elevator, walk up the stairs to your office. Pack a pair of sneakers in the car, park a mile or two away from your office, and walk the rest of the way. Take a walk during your lunch hour. Ride your bike to work when the weather permits. Get a group together and hire an aerobics teacher or a dance, yoga, or tai chi teacher to conduct a class in a conference room after work, before work, or during lunch hour. As the Nike ads say, "Just do it."

The goal of your exploration should be to find an exercise that is tolerable and that you can work into your weekly schedule on a regular basis. Although you probably won't love exercising at first, if you force yourself to stick with it, within a year you are likely to discover you've become addicted. After six months or so you'll begin to notice the salutary effects—a leaner, trimmer body, greater strength and energy, newfound emotional well-being, and a reduction in stress. Before many more months have passed, you may well find that you crave exercise and that when you don't get it you feel sluggish and cranky. Ironically, even at this point, it's easy to rationalize being lazy. But if you force yourself to get moving, those endorphins will surge, and you will feel revitalized.

LOSING WEIGHT AND KEEPING IT OFF

Millions of women, slim in their youth, helplessly watch themselves spread with age. Many try one fad diet after the next, only to fail. Some hope to eat whatever they want and exercise their weight away. This strategy also fails. But when they combine a low-fat eating style with regular exercise, their unwanted pounds miraculously begin to melt away. They automatically decrease their caloric intake as they reduce the fat in their diet, while their exercise program burns additional calories and raises their metabolism. As a result, they acquire a sense of control over their bodies and enjoy their first enduring weight loss. Even older women, whose metabolism naturally slows down, have found that combining diet and exercise works.

It stands to reason that a low-fat diet will help you lose weight permanently. Gram for gram, fats are the most fattening food. A gram of carbohydrate or pure protein contains four calories, while a gram of fat contains nine. Moreover, digesting and metabolizing carbohydrates takes more energy than metabolizing fats. Consequently, a diet rich in complex carbohydrates helps raise your metabolism. As several studies have shown, excess weight is tied to fat consumption, not caloric intake. Thus, few vegetarians are overweight. People who eat a diet rich in complex carbohydrates and very low in fat tend to lose weight effortlessly until their bodies find their best weight, determined largely by their genes.

If you don't find yourself losing one to two pounds a week as you cut back on fat and begin exercising regularly, reduce your fat intake more. Limit your visible fats to three units a day (1 unit = 1 teaspoon oil, margarine, or mayonnaise; 1½ teaspoons salad dressing; or 2 teaspoons reduced-fat mayonnaise) and your protein to a maximum of four ounces. If you still have trouble, you might consider working with a registered dietitian, who will help you design an effective and healthy weight-loss program tailored just for you.

Americans are the fattest people in the world, and obesity is clearly dangerous. According to the Nurses Health Study, the leaner you are, the healthier you will be. Although most of the leanest women in this study of over 115,000 also smoked, being thin appeared to protect the participants from heart disease. Those who were 30 percent or more overweight suffered three times the incidence of heart disease as those who were 5 percent underweight, and those of average weight were at one-third greater risk than the leanest women. This research did not look at whether the women carried their excess weight around their waists or below it. Like those in the study who were vulnerable to trouble, at least 25 percent of American women over the age of thirty-five weigh too much, and paring down would probably improve their health.

How much should you weigh? The answer is more complex than a number on a chart. Women gain weight as they age in a natural attempt to offset the loss of estrogen that occurs with menopause. A weak form of estrogen is produced in fat cells, enough to minimize the uncomfortable symptoms of menopause for some women. As Dr. Elizabeth Barrett-Connor observed, in societies where women are less obsessed with thinness, women seem to have less trouble with hot flashes and other menopausal miseries.

Moreover, because muscle weighs more than fat, lean women who are physically fit weigh more than lean women who are not. When Metropolitan Life revised its height and weight tables in 1983, they found that the healthiest Americans were heavier than in 1959, when the charts were first compiled, and the revised charts reflect an increase of five to ten pounds in most categories. In their 1990 Dietary Guidelines, the U.S. departments of Agriculture and Health and Human Services recommended even higher weights.

Your ideal weight is a range you and your doctor should arrive at taking into consideration your heredity, age, and proportion of lean body mass (muscle, bones, and internal organs) to fat. Calipers, which measure fat in inches, are as important as a scale. Active people need weight in the form of muscle to keep them going; being stick thin is unhealthy. When women lose too much weight, they tire easily or become listless. But for the great majority of women, being too thin is not the problem.

Now, let's talk turkey about losing weight and staying slim. Oprah Winfrey personifies the truth about dieting. On November 15, 1989, wearing size 10 Calvin Klein jeans, Oprah pulled a wagon filled with fat onto the stage to demonstrate all she had lost, and she vowed never to gain it back. As she recounted her triumph with a liquid diet and her willpower to sip soda water while her friends ate dinner, anyone who has sustained a substantial weight loss knew that Oprah's resolve would be short-lived. Sure enough, on November 5, 1990, Oprah, back up to a size 16 and growing, welcomed a panel of women who bemoaned a similar fate. One woman, who attempted to reduce her caloric intake instead of reducing the fat in her diet, discovered the truth about this hopeless approach to weight control: The less she ate, the lower her metabolism got, and the more she had to starve herself in order to continue losing. Another woman talked about her inability to keep up a daily two-hour exercise regimen. From one story to the next, one theme kept reemerging: Staying thin was unbearably punitive.

Unable to withstand relentless punishment, people typically give up, gain their weight back, get disgusted with themselves, and try again. This yo-yo dieting, in addition to being demoralizing, is unhealthy. It plays havoc with the metabolism, makes the next diet more frustrating, and wrecks self-esteem. For some women, regaining lost weight is the ultimate failure. Yo-yo dieting is also directly tied to heart disease. A thirty-year analysis of the Framingham population suggests that the practice can double the risk of developing heart disease and dying from it. As these investigators noted, it is easier to lose weight than keep it off, and more research must be dedicated to this important challenge.

If you want to keep off the weight you lose—a feat that only an estimated 5 percent of dieters accomplish—you must abandon the notion of diet, which implies something temporary, and be ready to change your eating habits and keep exercising regularly for life. And then you've got to learn how to take the punishment out of it: to make low-fat food choices that are satisfying, to eat small amounts frequently enough to keep from being hungry, to learn enough about making low-fat selections that you can take your new eating style on vacation and business trips, to parties, and out to restaurants. People who successfully lose weight and keep it off identify what part food plays in their life and they figure out how to meet the need without consuming the calories. One woman, who realized she was drinking three hundred empty calories in wine every night, saved the wine for special occasions. But every night, she drank soda water with lime out of a lovely goblet because she realized she enjoyed fondling the glass as much as tasting the wine. Another, who was accustomed to tasting frequently as she cooked, kept a bowl of celery sticks near the stove so she could munch on those instead. If you like picnics, don't stop having picnics just because you're cutting your calories. If you enjoy fine dining, set the table with cloth napkins and light some candles.

According to a study of 108 mostly middle-aged women who lost at least 20 percent of their weight and kept it off, there are four keys to success. One, these women gradually changed their eating habits, adopting everyday foods that were low in fat and refined sugars. But they occasionally splurged on treats to keep from feeling deprived. They did not rely on appetite suppressants, fasting regimens, or extremely restrictive diets. Two, they exercised regularly, at least thirty minutes three times a week. Three, they had good coping skills for managing stress. Instead of looking to escape by eating, sleeping, or wishing their problems away, they confronted their problems, worked out productive solutions, sought professional help as they needed it, and made good use of social support. Four, when they lost their weight, they felt content about their bodies, a sign of good self-esteem. Apparently, people have an easier time controlling their weight when their self-esteem is high, and repairing the self-esteem may be a valuable adjunct to a weight loss effort.

DO YOU NEED MEDICATION, TOO?

By exercising regularly, eating a low-fat diet, and losing excess weight, you may well be able to change your risk profile for heart disease from ominous to optimistic. Despite your best efforts, however, you may need some help from modern medicine.

USING MEDICATION AND SURGERY TO LOWER CHOLESTEROL

A low-fat diet plus regular exercise can be extremely effective in reducing your blood levels of cholesterol. And diet together with exercise is, without question, the best way to achieve the goal. But the goal is more important than the method. If diet alone does not enable you to reach your cholesterol goal after a six-month trial, you may have to add medication. Cholesterol-lowering agents can do wonders, but, again, they must supplement, not replace, a low-fat diet.

Like all drugs, the various preparations that lower cholesterol have advantages, limitations, and side effects that affect different patients in different ways. For many patients, the first choice has been niacin, sometimes called vitamin B$_3$. When taken in megadoses (between one and three grams a day), niacin becomes a potent drug that can lower LDL cholesterol and triglycerides while raising HDL cholesterol. Although niacin can be purchased without a prescription, when the drug is taken in large enough doses to modify cholesterol, patients must be monitored by a physician because serious side effects including abnormal heart rhythms, excessive blood sugar levels, ulcers, and liver problems can result. More commonly, niacin (in non-timed-released form) can cause hot flashes, rashes, itching, and abdominal discomfort, which make the treatment objectionable.

One of the newest and probably best drug available is lovastatin (Mevacor). Introduced in 1987, lovastatin is the first of a new classification of drugs, called *statins*, and is unprecedented in its effectiveness. In fact, research results published late in 1991 showed lovastatin to be the first single drug, combined with a low-fat diet, to successfully shrink atherosclerotic plaque. The effect of lovastatin was so striking that the study was halted ahead of schedule and participants taking a placebo were switched to Mevacor.

When the drug first came out, experts worried that it would cause serious side effects, notably cataracts, liver damage, and muscle inflammation. However, experience suggests that these concerns are unwarranted; serious side effects have been rare. Most patients have no trouble tolerating Mevacor at all. Still, the drug is expensive, it remains relatively new, and its long-term effects are therefore unknown. Consequently, physicians may not feel confident about prescribing Mevacor until their patients have tried more time-tested alternatives first.

Among the most frequently prescribed drugs is gemfibrozil (Lopid), This agent is particularly effective in lowering triglycerides and raising HDL cholesterol. It also lowers LDL and, in research, has been correlated with reduced rates of heart attacks. The drug can cause stomach upset, but it is generally well tolerated.

Also commonly prescribed are cholestyramine (Questran) and colestipol (Colestid). These lower the LDL, but may raise triglycerides, and they can produce intolerable side effects including stomach upset, vomiting, and bloating. In addition, they may prevent other medications from being absorbed. Consequently, scheduling doses can be tricky.

Probucol (Lorelco) has also been popular for lowering cholesterol largely because most people have no problem with its side effects. Although the drug works well to lower LDL levels, it appears to lower HDL as well.

When exceedingly high cholesterol stubbornly refuses to drop, even with medication combined with diligent diet, the problem can be managed surgically. The procedure, known as ileal bypass, entails making an incision in the abdomen and bypassing the bottom portion of the small intestine, where cholesterol from food and from the bile secreted from the liver is absorbed into the bloodstream. Unable to be absorbed, the cholesterol is excreted instead.

This is a radical measure and clearly a last resort. Patients who have had this procedure commonly complain of gas and diarrhea, sometimes forever. Less frequently, gallstones, kidney stones, and intestinal obstructions result. Nevertheless, for patients whose cholesterol puts them in substantial jeopardy, the procedure's benefits can outweigh its hazards. In one study, the men and women who had ileal bypass needed 62 percent fewer coronary bypass operations, 78 percent fewer repeat coronary bypass procedures, and 55 percent fewer balloon angioplasties than those in the comparison group.

Because high cholesterol raises risk of heart disease so significantly, scientists are always searching for new ways to combat it. For patients born without normal cholesterol receptors, a rare inherited condition causing cholesterol levels five times above normal and heart attacks sometimes by age ten, there is new hope on the horizon: gene therapy. In a multistep procedure that incorporates surgical removal of part of the liver, researchers hope to infuse the remaining liver with genes that would permit the normal formation of cholesterol receptors. The goal of this treatment is to lower cholesterol 50 percent, to a point where conventional therapy might be effective. Only a few hundred patients have cholesterol high enough to qualify them for the first clinical trials, which began in 1992. If these trials are successful, researchers hope that the results will be long-lasting and that the technique may someday evolve into standard treatment for patients with more run-of-the-mill varieties of high cholesterol.

Treating High Blood Pressure

Research suggests that if your blood pressure can be held at 140/90 or below, your risk for heart attack and stroke falls substantially. However, at what point high blood pressure should be treated is the subject of some controversy, since mild hypertension does not progress in any predictable way. Some studies suggest that treating mild hypertension will not prevent heart attacks and strokes. Other research shows that lowering blood pressure too much can cause the very problems treatment is designed to prevent. Since side effects of blood pressure medications can be severe, the balance of benefit and risk deserves attention on an individual basis.

In older people, high blood pressure is usually characterized by elevated systolic pressure—the first number in the blood pressure reading (reflecting the pressure in the arteries when the heart contracts) exceeds 160—and the diastolic pressure, the second number, stays at 95 or below. In June 1991, a study of five thousand people, 57 percent women and 14 percent black, documented for the first time that treating isolated systolic hypertension in older people (the average age in the study was seventy-two) pays off well. Based on the results of this five-year study, called the Systolic Hypertension in the Elderly Program (SHEP) and published in the *Journal of the American Medical Association*, the investigators estimated that treatment could prevent at least thirty strokes and twenty-five heart attacks for every one thousand people treated. In SHEP, patients were treated with a small dose of a mild diuretic, which can deplete the body of potassium and magnesium while increasing blood levels of sugar and uric acid. Some experts believe that newer antihypertensive medications, which do not cause these side effects, might be preferable, but research has not been done to support the belief.

Among the population at large, high blood pressure is usually caused by elevated diastolic pressure or the pressure in the arteries during the heart's relaxation phase. Virtually everyone agrees that a diastolic pressure above 105 must be treated. Most experts agree that treating diastolic pressure over 100 is beneficial. The National High Blood Pressure Education Program, which is credited with helping to lower the death rate from blood-pressure-induced disease by 54 percent since 1972, advocates prescribing medication when diastolic pressure exceeds 90. The 90 to 100 range is the subject of greatest controversy.

Blood pressure varies with a number of factors, including time of day, level of stress, and position. Sometimes people get high blood pressure just from the anxiety associated with visiting the doctor, a phenomenon known as "white coat hypertension." If your doctor finds that your blood pressure is high, it's important to verify that it is consistently high. Arrange to have your blood pressure tested several times, at varying times of the day, in both arms. Thanks to new technology called an *ambulatory blood pressure monitor*, this is now possible at home. The small, lightweight, computerized device, which is worn for twenty-four hours, measures and records the wearer's blood pressure every thirty minutes during waking hours and once an hour during sleep. The physician can then study the record to get an accurate idea of the patient's blood pressure pattern.

With an accurate assessment, you and your doctor will be able to decide whether you should take medication after considering your other risk factors, your overall health, and your ability to tolerate these drugs.

The calcium channel blockers, ACE inhibitors, and beta blockers used to treat coronary heart disease are effective for treating high blood pressure as well (see Chapter 5). Each drug has specific benefits, limitations, and side effects. Together they afford a variety of options to help your physician provide the most beneficial treatment with a minimum of side effects.

Dietary Supplements

Healthy people on a well-balanced diet seldom need multivitamin supplements. If you take a multivitamin, choose one that contains 100 percent of the recommended daily allowance (USRDA) of all essential vitamins and minerals, including fifteen milligrams of iron. You can feel safe buying a generic brand.

Beta carotene, the building block of vitamin A (found in such foods as carrots, spinach, and apricots), and vitamin E have been correlated with protection against strokes. But there is insufficient evidence to support taking dietary supplements of these vitamins. Similarly, although omega-3 fatty acids, found primarily in fish, protect against heart disease in several ways, there is no research to support taking fish oil capsules. Plan to get your omega-3 fatty acids from eating fish frequently.

Aspirin

Although ample research documents the merits of daily aspirin for women who have already had a heart attack, there is inadequate evidence to suggest that every woman should take aspirin daily as a preventive measure. The best research to date comes from the Nurses Health Study and documents only that taking "one through six aspirin per week appears to be associated with a reduced risk" of a first heart attack. Since long-term use of aspirin can cause upset stomachs, ulcers, and bleeding problems, and since research has not specified optimal dose, we cannot universally recommend taking aspirin to prevent a first heart attack. In individual cases, however, potential benefit might outweigh risk. Talk to your doctor about this option.

Antibiotics

You may be susceptible to bacterial endocarditis, an inflammation of the lining of the heart, if you have had valve surgery or have any of the following conditions: mitral valve prolapse with valvular regurgitation (that is, a murmur as well as a click), other valve dysfunctions, most congenital heart defects, an enlarged heart, or a previous case of bacterial endocarditis. Some congenital defects, benign heart murmurs, pacemakers, and bypass surgery do not increase susceptibility.

If your heart condition puts you at risk for endocarditis, you should take antibiotics before any dental or medical procedure likely to cause bleeding. Make sure all your physicians and dentists know about your heart condition so they can prescribe accordingly.

GIVING UP CIGARETTES

You don't need to be told *again* that smoking is bad. Undoubtedly you already know, and if you're like 80 percent of other smokers, you've also tried to stop. Keep trying!

Although smoking does feel good and taste good, and although it helps you keep your weight down, its dangers far outweigh its benefits. But these dangers begin to abate just as soon as you quit. Within days, your blood pressure will begin to drop, your heart rate will slow down, your coronary spasms will diminish, and your blood will carry more oxygen. Within four months, the oxygen level of your blood will be high enough to increase your energy and stamina by 16 percent. The benefits will continue to accrue steadily. If you decide to quit at age fifty, by the time you are sixty-five your risk of dying from heart disease will be cut in *half!*

Most people who quit did so on their own after a minimum of four failed efforts. The key to their ultimate success was a difference in inner motivation. Either they got disgusted with the way they smelled, they got tired of being social pariahs, they were frightened into quitting by ominous symptoms or a bad medical report card, or some other experience made them suddenly take notice. Whatever the catalyst, it triggered in them a passion to succeed that was stronger than their addiction.

Apparently, the smoking habit has two components: nicotine addiction and behavioral associations. If you can find the passion to quit, it will probably get you through the nicotine withdrawal. While most former smokers simply quit cold turkey without help of any kind, some have found hypnosis and acupuncture eased them through this stage. Nicotine gum, which provides nicotine without the other harmful chemicals in cigarettes, can also help you overcome withdrawal symptoms. Although the gum can be addicting itself, people usually have less difficulty weaning themselves from this crutch than from the cigarettes. Nicotine gum is available with a doctor's prescription, and it must be used according to specific directions. (Research has suggested ordinary chewing gum may work as well.)

What about the skin patch that delivers a trickle of nicotine into the bloodstream over a twenty-four-hour period? Like nicotine gum, the patch helps to ease only the physical aspect of the addiction. Managing the psychological side requires strong motivation and possibly the assistance of counseling, a support group, motivational tapes, or the like. According to a University of Nebraska study, people who relied on the patch were about as successful as those who quit cold turkey—about 26 percent. Some people have found the patches irritate their skin. A few have reported side effects such as abdominal pain, rapid heartbeat, bizarre dreams, insomnia, and sweating. And the patches are expensive: about $120 a month.

Separate from purging your body of the nicotine addiction, you need to dissociate yourself and your activities from cigarettes. If you normally smoke at the table after dinner, get up when the meal is over and go for a walk. If you habitually smoke at your desk, munch on carrot sticks instead. Chew gum. Sip herbal tea. Take walks. Brush your teeth. Step outside, breathe deeply, and enjoy the sensation of filling your lungs with air. Call a friend who also quit and complain. Call a friend who still smokes and boast. Instead of thinking that you will never smoke again, think about one day at a time. Save the money you would ordinarily spend on cigarettes and plan an extravagance. Set yourself some modest goals and, as you achieve each one, reward your success with a make-over, manicure, or some other treat.

If you feel you would benefit from guidance and peer support, call your local chapter of the American Lung Association, the American Cancer Society, or the American Heart Association to learn about local programs to quit smoking. These will teach you the techniques of behavior modification and provide the encouragement and empathy of others who have taken on the same difficult challenge.

If you relapse, pick yourself up, brush yourself off, and start all over again. You can't succeed if you don't try.

REDUCING STRESS

Stress—distress, rather—causes a series of biochemical events that have profound effects on health. Stress alters immunity to infection, increases acid in the stomach and causes ulcers, and harms the heart. Stress hormones raise blood pressure, increase heart rate, and damage the lining of the coronary arteries, thereby inviting blood clots and plaque formation. The antithesis to this stress response is a condition that Harvard cardiologist Herbert Benson, M.D., termed the *relaxation response.* In the absence of stress, we are better able to fight off infection. Ulcers heal, migraine headaches go away, heart rate and blood pressure settle down.

Although living in a state of relaxation is healthier, stress is part of the American life-style. The challenge, then, is to mediate stress to diminish its ill effects. Before you can cope with stress, however, you have to be able to recognize it. If your stomach turns in knots and you start to sweat in anticipation of giving a speech, you're not likely to overlook the sensation. Or if you're under a deadline and your head seems to pound with the ticking of the clock, again, your stress is apparent. But sometimes we hunch our shoulders or clench our teeth in response to chronic or subtle stress without even being aware of it, and these behaviors reflect more pernicious stress reactions going on inside.

Experts recommend making a conscious effort to analyze your stress response. Hunch up your shoulders and then relax them. Tighten your jaw, then relax it. Pay attention to the differences in feeling. Check your posture as you pass a mirror. Stop what you're doing periodically and note your level of tension. Train yourself to recognize the difference between tense and relaxed muscles. Keep an activity diary for a day or so to record when tension arises and see if you can chart a pattern. Once you have a clear sense of when you feel stress and what's causing it, you can take steps to alleviate it, or, as psychologists like to phrase it, you can modify your behavior.

Eliminate the Source of Stress

Typically, stress comes from feeling out of control. We're late for a meeting and we're stuck in traffic. We have a deadline and not enough time to get the work done. Obviously, one way to recapture control is by identifying the problem and solving it. If you feel over-burdened by too many volunteer commitments or unrelenting demands from family or friends, learn to say no. If you tend to become overwhelmed by having too much to do and too little time, try to avoid imposing unrealistic expectations on yourself. Set priorities. Abandon unimportant tasks. Break down the large jobs into more manageable components and focus on one at a time. Make lists and cross off your accomplishments one by one. Avoid the tendency to set unrealistic goals; if you try to accomplish more than time reasonably allows, you set a trap for frustration. Conversely, if you can avoid imposing unrealistic expectations on yourself, you will have an easier time maintaining a sense of control.

If you have a chronic tendency to feel pressed for time, figure out how you can give yourself more time. When you schedule your day, allow for delays, interruptions, phone calls. If you are a procrastinator, make a concerted effort to start your projects early. If crowds and long lines make you crazy, don't wait to do your Christmas shopping until December 23. We can avoid many of life's stresses by breaking overwhelming tasks into manageable components, managing our time effectively, and employing other problem-solving strategies.

Control Your Perception

Psychologists tell a tall tale about testing identical twins, one an optimist and one a pessimist. The pessimist was placed in a light, bright room filled with interesting diversions and told to have fun. The optimist was placed in a room filled with manure and given a shovel. Two hours later, the pessimist was found sitting in the corner feeling dejected and complaining that, among all the diversions, she couldn't find her favorite computer chess game. The optimist was found happily shoveling away. When asked what she was doing, the optimist replied, "With all this horse dung, there's got to be a pony in here somewhere."

As the story suggests, it is always possible to see the proverbial glass as half full, not half empty. When stress is unavoidable, a positive attitude may not change the situation, but it can enable you to control your reaction to it. In this way, optimism ameliorates frustration, hostility, and cynicism, all of which have been correlated to heart disease.

If you are forced to spend a boring, tiring day in the airport because your flight has been canceled, you could obsess about the appointments you have to reschedule or the party you'll miss or the time you're wasting or the boredom you're feeling. Or you could turn your fate into a positive experience. Instead of seething or brooding, get absorbed in people watching. Or study how couples relate to each other. Or try to analyze the marketing strategies of the airport vendors. Or buy the kind of book or magazine you never get the time to read and lose yourself in it. Or take advantage of the opportunity for exercise and walk from one end of the concourse to the other.

Stuck in traffic? Find your local National Public Radio station, usually in the vicinity of 90 FM, and get absorbed in some of their fascinating programs. Or carry some of your own favorite music tapes in the car for just this eventuality. If you anticipate spending a long, frustrating time in the car, consider borrowing a book on tape from your library and catching up on your "reading." Plan a project or think through the solution to a problem; keep a tape recorder in the car so you can make note of your ideas. If you use your time productively, the minutes will pass and you'll hardly even know it.

While we can't always control our emotions completely, we can often ameliorate them by reasoning them away. The next time you sense negative emotions brewing, try to analyze what's causing them. Intellectually speaking, is whatever you're stewing about really worth the emotional energy it's producing? Permit your intellectual self to shake your emotional self by the shoulders, and some of your negative feelings are likely to subside. Don't brood; if you can't do something constructive to change a situation, try to dismiss it from your mind. Employing a positive attitude and emotionally detaching yourself from difficult circumstances help defuse unavoidable stress and the feelings of frustration, anger, and cynicism it generates.

Because stress is so pernicious, stress management has been the subject of enduring exploration. In addition to behavior modification, a number of other effective techniques have been developed.

Biofeedback

Biofeedback trains people to recognize their physiological responses to the world. The technique, which utilizes sensitive technology to record changes in body temperature, blood pressure, brain waves, and other physiological factors, is based on the premise that if people become conscious of body processes once considered involuntary, they can influence those processes. Biofeedback raises people's awareness of the physiological responses their emotions produce and thus helps them recognize stress so that they can ameliorate it with another technique, such as meditation, self-hypnosis, or progressive relaxation.

Meditation

Meditation, including transcendental meditation, Chakra yoga, Rinzai Zen, Mudra yoga, Sufism, Zen meditation, and Soto Zen, is one of the most widely used mental exercises that affects physiological processes. By meditating for twenty minutes twice a day, people control what they concentrate on, rather than being bombarded by stimuli around them. This concentration brings inner peace, which, in turn, slows respiration and heart rate, decreases muscle tension, reduces anxiety, and enhances feelings of psychological well-being. While these effects are most pronounced while people are meditating, research shows they carry over to the rest of the day.

Meditation and the yoga exercises that sometimes accompany it require detailed instruction and some practice before you can expect them to work for you. You can get a sense of the experience, however, with the following exercises. Try them both, select the one you prefer or which seems to work best, or use them alternately.

- Find a comfortable, quiet place where you can sit undisturbed. Concentrate on breathing deeply, slowly, and regularly in through the nose and out through the mouth. Each time you exhale, repeat the word "one" . . . "one" . . . "one."
- Breathe deeply, slowly, and regularly, imagine blowing your anxiety away each time you exhale. Like a balloon, it sails away, rises up, and disappears.

Your goal with these exercises is to focus your attention so acutely that you become oblivious of everything else around you. At that point, you should be in a state of total relaxation. Try to sustain it for twenty minutes.

Self-hypnosis

Unlike meditation, which uses the mind to relax the body, self-hypnosis uses the physical sensations to relax the body, and then, in turn, the mind. In the hypnotic state, the blood vessels dilate, producing a sensation of warmth, and the muscles relax, making the arms and legs feel heavy. People induce this state by concentrating on sensations of warmth and coolness as well as lightness and heaviness in one area of the body after the next. Although self-hypnosis requires substantial motivation and far more practice than meditation, it produces comparable results. Observations first noted around the turn of the century suggest that the technique reduces fatigue, tension, and headaches. More recent research documents that it moderates anxiety and depression while it helps people resist stress.

One part of the self-hypnotic process involves imaging. While the entire process does require instruction and practice, you can get a sense of what it's about with the following imaging exercises. As with meditation, choose a quiet place and a comfortable position. Try to sustain a state of relaxation for twenty minutes.

- Breathing deeply, slowly, and regularly, transport yourself mentally to a beautiful and peaceful place: a quiet Caribbean cove, a silent forest, a peaceful mountaintop.
- Breathing slowly and regularly, take yourself through a series of images: a tropical jungle dense with dewy green; the chirping of birds high in the pines of Montana woods; the sweet fragrance of lilacs; the taste of ice cream, smooth and cold.

Progressive Relaxation

Progressive relaxation teaches people to recognize the difference between tense and relaxed muscles so they can make their muscles relax on command. Concentrating on one muscle group at a time, participants tense up and then let go in an attempt to relax the entire body. As in self-hypnosis, this physical relaxation then extends to the mind. Studies show that the relaxation one achieves in relaxing the muscles of the skeleton spread to the smooth muscles of the intestinal and cardiovascular systems. The technique also helps to alleviate headaches, backaches, and other psychosomatic symptoms while reducing depression and anxiety and raising feelings of self-esteem. The following is a progressive relaxation exercise:

- Lying comfortably on your back, tense your feet and relax them. Squeeze and let go; squeeze, let go, and let them lie limp. Then do the same three times with your leg muscles followed by your other muscles in sequence: your hands, your arms, your buttocks, your abdomen, your chest, your jaw, your face. By the time you are finished, your entire body should be relaxed. Try and sustain your relaxed state for twenty minutes.

Coping with stress is a highly personal matter. Some people take to conscious relaxation techniques quickly and discover that periods of imposed calm are surprisingly refreshing. Others must make a concerted effort to force relaxation when their head is bursting and their body feels tense. But they have enough motivation to get instruction and practice until the skill becomes useful. Nearly everyone who practices conscious relaxation prefers one technique to another, and some people simply feel conscious relaxation of any kind is hokey or alien to their personalities or, ironically, stress-producing. If conscious relaxation works for you, great. If not, there are other options. No matter what strategy you choose, give yourself the gift of stress relief.

Take Advantage of Emotional Support

Recent research by Duke University's Redford Williams, M.D., who discovered that anger and hostility are the most pernicious components of the Type A behavior pattern, revealed that love and friendship are critical to surviving heart disease. Research by Georgetown University's Deborah Tannen, Ph.D., suggests that women are particularly adept at using close relationships to vent their emotions, acquire empathy and support, and otherwise experience the salutary effects of love and friendship. Reach out to those who love you, and when they reach out to you, accept their embrace. (For more on emotional support, see Chapter 8.)

Rely on Exercise and Relaxation

Because exercise raises your levels of endorphins, hormones that dull pain and elevate mood, it is an effective safety valve for stress. Use exercise to purge yourself of stress. If you feel pressured during the workday, try to get out for a brisk walk at lunchtime. When tension mounts, vent it physically: Pull weeds in the garden, walk the dog, wash the car. During particularly busy or stressful periods, make a concerted effort to save some time to work out.

One way or another, reserve some time for yourself. You deserve —no, you need (everyone needs)—to spend time doing whatever soothes your soul. Lie in a dark room and listen to music. Go window-shopping. Light a candle and soak in a bubble bath. Get a massage or a manicure or a facial. Take a walk in the woods. Spend a contemplative moment in church or synagogue. Whatever you choose, the time you spend on yourself is time well spent because it will replenish your coping reserves and help you function more effectively.

Get Professional Help

If you find you cannot manage your stress on your own, consider getting some help from the experts. Professionally guided support groups, individual counseling, and various workshops in stress management have helped many, many people acquire a badly needed sense of control. To find help in your community, call your local mental health association for a reputable referral.

PROTECTING YOUR CHILDREN'S HEALTH

Children under the age of two need a diet rich in fat. Medical researchers discovered this truth when a group of health-conscious Long Island mothers inadvertently stunted their toddlers' growth by feeding them skim milk. Between ages two and three, children's fat needs are in transition. By the time they are three years old, however, children's diets, like their parents', should contain a maximum of 30 percent fat.

Beginning at age two, it is important to shape children's taste for low-fat foods. If they resist, help them make the transition gradually. Mix whole milk with 2 percent fat milk at first, and then increase the proportion of 2 percent. Continue gradually reducing the fat content until they're drinking skim milk. Switch from whole eggs to predominantly egg whites. To increase their fiber, accustom your children to whole-grain breads, brown rice, and other grains.

If they love fried chicken, skin chicken legs, dip them in egg white, roll them in crumbs made from crushed Shredded Wheat cereal; bake on a cookie sheet coated with cooking oil spray at 450° for forty minutes or until they're cooked. Make fish sticks from a mild white fish, such as cod or halibut, in a similar way; bake one-inch sticks at 500° for ten minutes. Make lots and have them on hand in the freezer for a quick supper or lunch. Make sure that the frozen kiddie fare you buy contains no more than three grams of fat for every one hundred calories. Use peanut butter as a substitute for other protein, not as a snack. Give your kids bagels and pretzels instead of cookies, unbuttered popcorn instead of chips.

Make a special effort to avoid programming your children to eat except when they are hungry. When they say they're full, let them stop eating. If they seem uninterested in food, let them not eat. They won't starve. If parents use something other than food for rewards and punishments, perhaps the children will grow up with less difficulty controlling their weight.

Talk to your pediatrician about whether your children should have their cholesterol tested. While keeping children over three on a low-fat diet is unquestionably a good idea, there is some controversy about whether it's an equally good idea to have their cholesterol tested. Some research suggests that high cholesterol tends to resolve itself as children grow older. According to a study of over two thousand youngsters age eight to eighteen, most children, even those with the highest numbers, did not need cholesterol-lowering treatment by the time they reached age thirty. Perhaps this trend reflects a change in eating patterns over time. Perhaps it is a natural by-product of growth and development. Regardless, the experts at the National Cholesterol Education Program feel that widespread screening is more than unwarranted; it may result in children being labeled with a disease they might never get and suffering all the anxiety that can accompany such a designation. The National Cholesterol Education Program recommends testing children only if one of their parents has cholesterol over 240 or atherosclerosis or heart disease tends to strike the family before age fifty-five.

Make sure your daughters are getting enough calcium, especially during their teenage years, so that they build skeletal equity for their later years. Girls need 800 milligrams of calcium until they are ten years old and 1,200 milligrams from age eleven to age twenty-four.

Help your children realize early in life how good it feels to have a strong and agile body. Sign them up for soccer teams, gymnastics sessions, martial arts, swimming lessons. Make sure their after-school and day-care programs provide lots of opportunity for running, climbing, and sports. According to research published in January 1992, kids are a lot less active today than young people used to be. This nationwide survey of nearly 12,000 high school students showed that only 37 percent exercise vigorously for twenty minutes or more three times a week. This number is down from 62 percent in 1984. The decline among girls was a shocking 75 percent, compared to 50 percent among the boys, and the worst offenders were the twelfth-grade girls: Only 17 percent said they exercise regularly.

The habits kids establish today may last their whole lives, so turn off the television and get those kids outside. Aside from all the merits of exercise, children who watch television for two hours or more a day tend to have high cholesterol, a study of over one thousand

youngsters ages two to twenty revealed. These young people probably eat junk while they watch and get insufficient exercise. In addition, commercials for junk food undoubtedly sabotage Mother's
preference for buying and serving healthful fare.

When it comes to taking care of your children, as with reducing
your own stress, modifying your diet and living a heart-smart way in
every other respect, you are in charge. Take on the challenge. Accept
the responsibility. Work with your doctor. And enjoy how good you
will look and feel.

EPILOGUE
Assuring a Healthier Tomorrow

In October 1991, Anita Hill filed sexual harassment charges against Clarence Thomas, then-nominee for Supreme Court justice, and an all-male Senate Judiciary Committee presumed that they could find truth. "The absence on the [Senate Judiciary] panel of anyone who could become pregnant accidentally or discover that her salary was $5,000 a year less than that of her male counterpart meant there was a hole in the consciousness of the committee that empathy, however welcome, could not entirely fill," wrote Anna Quindlen in *The New York Times*. "The need for more women in elective office was vivid every time the cameras panned that line of knotted ties."

Similarly, a male dominance in medicine has assured a male perspective in every facet of the profession, from medical school classes to clinical practices and the allocation of research funds. One reason why women's health has been ignored is that there are few female medical researchers, especially in senior positions. Researchers tend to study issues that concern them. As an editorial in *Science for All America* noted, when male scientists studied the social behavior of primates, they concentrated on the competitive behavior of males. The importance of the primates' community-building activities, which is a female behavior, was not recognized until women began doing the research. A larger body of female medical scientists is likely to assure increased attention to women's health and investigations designed to detect the differences between the sexes. Encourage your daughters and granddaughters to pursue careers in medical research.

By the same token, it's women's job to keep female health issues at the forefront of public consciousness. While attitudes toward women's health have begun to change, progress will continue only if that awareness remains alive. Several advocacy groups have begun working toward this end. In February 1990, the Society for the Advancement of Women's Health Research, located at 1601 Connecticut Avenue, N.W., Suite 801, Washington, D.C. 20001 (202-328-2200), was established to promote the cause, with particular attention to women of color, older women, and women with specific medical conditions. In the fall of 1990, the Jacobs Institute of Women's Health was founded by the American College of Obstetrics and Gynecology to bring relevant social issues to the awareness of health professionals. Also that fall the Office of Research in Women's Health was opened at the NIH to coordinate research on women among the various institutes.

Do your part. Affiliate with one of the more than forty organizations that support the Campaign for Women's Health. This coalition, formed with initial funding of the Ms. Foundation, was organized in 1991 to help define the problems contributing to inequities in health care; propose solutions; and provide leadership, advocacy, and technical backup to effect those solutions. The Campaign for Women's Health is a project of the Older Women's League and is supported by diverse organizations, among them the American Association of University Women, Black Women's Agenda, B'Nai B'Rith Women, Catholics for a Free Choice, National Foundation for Women Business Owners, National Organization for Women, National Women's Health Network, and the YWCA. Join one of the supporting organizations and help keep this issue alive. To learn more about this growing coalition and its work, contact the Campaign for Women's Health at 666 Eleventh Street, N.W., Suite 700, Washington, D.C. 20001 (202-738-6686).

Support the legislators responsible for the inroads made to date, including Representatives Henry Waxman, Pat Schroeder, and Olympia Snowe; Senators Barbara Mikulski, Edward Kennedy, and Tom Harkin. The more women in political office, the greater the assurance that women's health will continue to get the attention and the funding it needs. Make this issue a campaign point in your district, and support the candidates, male and female, who are sympathetic to it.

On a personal level, practice heart-smart habits to set a good example for your family while you take care of yourself. The mother who eats well probably serves healthful meals and helps her children acquire healthy tastes early in life. And the mother who works out regularly lets her children know that exercise is an important priority. These children are likely to grow up with habits that will keep them healthy throughout their lives.

Pay attention to what's going on in school. Are physical education classes nurturing a love of exercise? Do your kids have the opportunity to run around during recess? Is your child's school promoting good nutrition in the classroom and the cafeteria? Persuading the school to foster healthy habits is an ideal way to teach your children about speaking out and effecting change.

Women hold tremendous power to shape the health and habits of others. Women are legislators and researchers, physicians and teachers. They are nurses and nutritionists, shoppers and cooks. As policy makers, caretakers, and nurturers, women are in a unique position to make a difference—for themselves, for their families, and for generations to come.

AFTERWORD

In chapter 1, we spoke with outrage about the pervasive ignorance surrounding heart disease as the primary killer of women. If we were writing that chapter now, we might well take a less strident tone. Just one year since *Women and Heart Disease* first went to press, women and men across the country have become suddenly aware of the issue, and interest is keen. It has been an active and important year for developments in research and public policy as well. As the paperback edition goes to press, we are delighted to have this opportunity to bring you up to date.

Antioxidant Vitamins: No sooner had the manuscript left our hands for the last time than several studies fortified the growing belief that taking antioxidant vitamins may help to ward off coronary heart disease, as well as certain kinds of cancer. According to two studies presented first at the American Heart Association scientific meetings in November 1992 and then published in *The New England Journal of Medicine* the following May, daily doses of vitamin E cut the risk of heart disease substantially. In one report, gleaned from the long-running Nurses' Health Study of over 87,000 women, those who took at least 100 international units of vitamin E daily for at least two years showed a 46 percent lower rate of heart attack. The other data, from the Harvard School of Public Health Study of nearly 52,000 men, showed a 37 percent reduction. The most compelling data to date, these findings strengthen the conclusions of several earlier studies suggesting that vitamins E, C, and beta carotene (a building block of vitamin A) might be therapeutic.

Here's how antioxidants work: Ordinarily, the oxygen we breathe is used to fuel cells throughout the body. In the process, a waste product called free radicals, or oxidants, is released. According to the antioxidant theory, these free radicals serve as catalysts to the atherosclerotic process (see chapter 2). Vitamins E, C, and beta carotene appear to prevent the catalytic action of free radicals, thereby slowing or stopping the formation of plaque on the artery walls.

Although the new findings are compelling, they are incomplete. Until controlled clinical trials are performed, there is no way to know whether what appears to be cause and effect is, in fact, cause and effect. Even if the correlation is valid, important questions remain. For starters, if taking vitamin supplements proves to be beneficial, what is the ideal dose, and what is the downside of taking megadoses of these vitamins for many years? More definitive information will be available by the end of the decade, with the conclusion of several large studies of women and men.

Until then, whether you should take supplements of these vitamins and what dosages you should take are decisions to be discussed with your physician. Certainly, eating generous portions of foods that contain these vitamins is a good idea, especially since most of them are consistent with a low-fat, high-fiber diet. Foods rich in vitamin E include fortified cereals, wheat germ, brown rice, kale, lettuce, dried apricots, and sunflower and pumpkin seeds. Foods rich in vitamin C include citrus fruits, papaya, tomatoes, cantaloupe, clams, green pepper, kiwi, and broccoli. Good sources of beta carotene include carrots, sweet potatoes, yellow squash, spinach, and cantaloupe.

Iron: In chapter 10, you read about the importance of getting adequate iron in the diet. In late 1992, however, headlines suggested that excessive iron might actually cause heart disease. The research at issue, a study out of Finland published in *Circulation* in September 1992, found that iron-rich blood more than doubles the risk of heart attacks in men. So strong was the finding that an accompanying editorial suggested that iron might prove to be a more potent risk factor than cholesterol.

The Finnish researchers theorized that iron, although needed in small amounts to prevent anemia, might foster the formation of free radicals. Perhaps, they hypothesized, women of childbearing age have less heart disease not because they are protected by estrogen but because they lose iron in their monthly menstrual blood.

By March 1993, three additional studies had thrown the results of this one into question, and today the iron issue remains unresolved. Nevertheless, the Finnish study is important if only because it reminds us how easy it is to jump to premature conclusions, in this case, about why young women are protected from heart disease. We presume without irrefutable proof that the protector is estrogen, and then along comes research that says, "maybe not."

Whether or not excess iron proves to be a risk factor, the very theory reinforces the conviction that most Americans eat too much red meat and that it's more than safe to cut back. If you want to further hedge your bets, give blood.

Cholesterol: A number of provocative studies on cholesterol and how to keep it in line have been published since this book first went to press. The most intriguing research, published in Circulation in September 1992, was accompanied by an editorial calling for a change in policy on managing cholesterol levels.

One surprising report—actually a pooled analysis of 125,000 men and women from twenty-four studies with follow-up periods of up to thirty years—showed that high cholesterol in women does not—repeat, does not—correlate to death from any cause, cardiovascular diseases included, although the predicted correlation does occur in men. This finding is shocking, especially since we know that high cholesterol does increase women's risk for heart disease, and heart disease is the number one cause of death.

Perhaps the explanation lies in the study design. Data were analyzed after grouping heart attacks together with other cardiovascular diseases, strokes caused by bleeding (as well as strokes caused by blood clots) among them. Separate research has shown that as cholesterol goes down, risk of hemorrhagic stroke goes up. The net result appears to be a statistical peculiarity: In women, as well as in men, risk of hemorrhagic stroke is relatively rare. Since women also experience a low rate of heart disease in middle age, the small number of deaths from strokes may offset the number of deaths from heart attacks.

This finding was published in the "Report of the Conference on

Low Blood Cholesterol: Mortality Associations." Another mortality association reported by the conference was an increase in premature deaths from causes other than cardiovascular disease when cholesterol levels fall below 160. Men and women with very low cholesterol —these people account for approximately 6 percent of the population—are excessively vulnerable to death from such causes as cancer, respiratory disease, digestive disease, and trauma.

On the basis of both these findings, Stephen Hulley and his co-authors, who wrote the accompanying editorial, questioned the merits of nationwide policy devoted to lowering everyone's cholesterol. They recommend screening women's cholesterol and treating their high cholesterol with drugs only if women have a very high risk profile or established cardiovascular disease. This recommendation, or course, reflects a radical departure from the National Cholesterol Education Program's existing policy, which, unfortunately, was created by extrapolating male data to women.

It's important to note that the editorial, in addressing public policy, attempts to balance known benefit against potential risk and cost for the population at large. Public policy is very different from the recommendation any one physician makes to any one patient. Whether your risk profile (see chapter 3) warrants regular screening and your high cholesterol needs treatment with medication is something you must discuss with your physician.

While the editorial questions the wisdom of treating elevated cholesterol aggressively with medication, it does not suggest abandoning healthful eating or exercise habits. Heart disease is, after all, a killer to contend with. Regular exercise and a diet low in fat and high in fiber are mighty weapons.

The following March, Dr. Hulley published another article, this one in the *Journal of the American Medical Association*, recommending that the National Cholesterol Education Program stop advising young adults to know their cholesterol. Dr. Hulley argues that high cholesterol alone is a poor predictor of actual heart disease and that disease is rare among young people. Since most benefits of cholesterol treatment occur when treatment begins at a later age and since we have no way to predict the damage that might result from taking cholesterol-lowering medication for many years, Dr. Hulley advises withholding screening until men reach thirty-five and women forty-five. By not screening the 80 million younger American adults, billions of health care dollars would be saved.

Not surprisingly, the article generated substantial controversy. Supporting Dr. Hulley's position, several experts pointed to the observation that maximum benefit occurs in the first two years of treating cholesterol, so it makes sense to begin treatment when risk of developing disease becomes significant. In fact, a Canadian task force recommended abandoning cholesterol screening of young adults in 1990. However, advocates of the existing National Cholesterol Education Program point to the truth that coronary artery disease is a cumulative process that begins early in life and that slowing the process can have profound effects.

Again, the issue seems to be the cost-benefit ratio of massive screening and the potential risk associated with relying on drugs prematurely. No one is refuting the fact that high cholesterol raises heart attack risk. Nor is anyone arguing the merit of healthy diet and regular exercise, which help keep cholesterol low and health good.

Hormone Replacement Therapy: The merits of taking hormone replacement to protect the heart and the bones have become so convincing that the American College of Physicians devoted one of its Guideline series to the subject in December 1992. In the Guidelines, a regular feature of the *Annals of Internal Medicine,* the College has traditionally presented a review of the available research on a particular subject together with didactic advice to practicing clinicians.

The College chose hormone replacement for the Guideline series because, despite irrefutable evidence that estrogen protects the heart and the bones, the FDA has yet to approve estrogen for any purpose other than relieving the symptoms of menopause. The authors of the review article concluded, "Hormone therapy should probably be recommended for women who have had a hysterectomy and for those with coronary heart disease or at high risk for coronary heart disease. For other women, the best course of action is unclear." Despite this apparent equivocation—necessary because of lingering questions, specifically about the role of progesterone and increased risk of breast cancer—the college refrained from taking a didactic position.

Recognizing that women have different risk factors and different value systems, the College instead decided to lay out the benefits and risks so that physicians could help each of their patients choose what is medically sound and emotionally comfortable for her. This is a striking departure from previous practice.

For the first time in its history, the College advocated that its physicians make clinical decisions in partnership with their patients. How interesting that this change was initiated in the context of women's health, particularly in an area that remains controversial and that generates such passion.

It is also noteworthy that, despite an absence of data on starting hormone replacement many years after menopause, the Guidelines state "beginning treatment in older women may also be beneficial."

The following April, a study published in *The New England Journal of Medicine* helped strengthen the notion that progesterone, taken with estrogen to protect the uterus from endometrial cancer (see chapter 9), might also help protect the heart. In this observational study of nearly 5,000 women, those who took estrogen plus a progesterone like Provera had a healthier risk profile for heart disease than women who took estrogen alone. This study, whose population was racially and geographically diverse, suggests that progesterone does not interfere with estrogen's ability to improve cholesterol and has the added benefit of lowering triglycerides and certain blood clotting factors. Because this is an observational study, not a clinical trial, it is not definitive. Numerous questions remain, among them what the ideal dosage of progesterone should be. Nevertheless, in an accompanying editorial, Kathryn Martin, M.D., and Mason Freeman, M.D., acknowledging that progesterone might help prevent osteoporosis as well, recommended that when the uterus is intact and women take hormone therapy to protect their hearts, they should take a progestin for at least ten days a month.

The fact that Drs. Martin and Freeman make this recommendation and that it was published in *The New England Journal of Medicine* is noteworthy. In the past, as the recent Guidelines issued by the American College of Physicians reflect, prudent thinkers have refrained from advocating progesterone when hormone replacement was prescribed to protect the heart because there was some reason to believe that progesterone might mitigate the beneficial effects of estrogen. In any event, not enough was known about the impact of progesterone to warrant recommending it. Over the past several years, bits of evidence have begun to suggest that progesterone was not harmful and might even help protect the heart (see chapter 9). In light of Drs. Martin's and Freeman's editorial, we can conclude that this study substantially advances the theory that progesterone is protective.

Results of the GUSTO Trial: In chapter 6, we reported on the controversy surrounding two drugs used to dissolve blood clots in the hours immediately following a heart attack. At issue were streptokinase and tPA, a genetically engineered alternative that costs at least ten times more. Although most American medical centers have been using tPA because preliminary studies suggested it is a superior drug, a huge international study published in March 1992 showed that streptokinase works as well. The debate, we said in chapter 6, would be resolved finally with the results of the GUSTO trial, and these results have now been published.

In the GUSTO, or Global Utilization of Streptokinase and tPA, trial, 41,000 heart attack patients in fifteen countries participated in random testing of four regimens. One group received intravenous tPA together with aspirin and heparin (another clot-dissolving medication). A second group received streptokinase plus aspirin and intravenous heparin. A third group received streptokinase, as well as aspirin and heparin under the skin. And the fourth group received both tPA and streptokinase, plus aspirin and heparin. After thirty days, patients who received tPA, heparin, and aspirin within ninety minutes of attack were least likely to die (6.3 percent death rate), followed by streptokinase combined with tPA (7.0 percent), followed by the two streptokinase regimens (7.2 percent and 7.4 percent respectively). These results translate to a 14 percent advantage for tPA—small but significant.

Weighing the size of the tPA advantage against the cost of the drug poses a real dilemma, particularly in the context of today's health care crisis. Perhaps the most important evidence to come from this study, however, is conclusive proof that rapid dissolution of clots does save lives. This finding underscores a point we make in chapter 6: In the United States, more heart attack patients need to be treated more quickly with clot-dissolving drugs. Which drug is chosen is secondary.

Developments in Health Policy: We closed chapter 1 with fingers crossed, hoping that the health care crisis and money crunch would not impede the long-overdue progress toward better health for all women. It is gratifying to report that, although Bernadine Healy no longer heads the National Institute of Health, the work she began there will continue. The recently passed NIH Reauthorization Act assures the permanence of the Office of Research on Women's Health, earmarks (but does not allocate) $500 million for women's health research, and mandates that all grants receiving NIH funds meet particular gender-specific guidelines.

The awareness spawned at the beginning of the decade has engendered substantial action and reaction. The NIH Reauthorization Act is a striking case in point. Feeling the urgent need to right the wrongs of discrimination against women in medical research, Congress proposed that all NIH funded clinical trials include sufficient women and minorities to permit separate analysis of the data for each subgroup. While this proposal sounds reasonable and appropriate, J. Claude Bennett, M.D., writing on behalf of the National Academy of Sciences, argued in a special report published in *The New England Journal of Medicine* that the proposal, as designed, is scientifically unsound, unnecessarily costly, and counterproductive to its purpose. We are heartened to see debate raging, for debate itself is a catalyst for critical thinking and the ideas it generates.

The FDA took action against sexism this year by changing its policies on including women in trials of new drugs. In the past, fear of birth defects and resulting liability led the FDA to keep women of childbearing age from the early phases of drug trials, even if they were sexually inactive or using reliable birth control. The FDA, acknowledging that this policy was unabashedly paternalistic, vows that women will be appropriately represented in clinical studies and threatens to reject applications that do not comply.

Heart disease in women dominated the annual scientific meetings of the American College of Cardiology in March 1993 and was the subject of a special article in the July 22 issue of *The New England Journal of Medicine*. This report, based on the proceedings of a National Heart, Lung, and Blood Institute conference held in January 1992, provided a comprehensive summary of heart disease in women, including recommendations for diagnosis, treatment, risk reduction, and research. In addition, the authors called for incorporating information about prevention and treatment into standard medical school curricula and postgraduate residency programs and making this subject a regular feature at medical professional meetings for virtually any physician who provides primary care to females—pediatricians included.

Finally, it is reassuring to report that the advocacy organizations we introduced in the Epilogue have made tangible gains protecting women's health in both the research and policy. The Society for the Advancement of Women's Health Research (see p. 268), which was founded in 1990 solely to overcome egregious sexism in medical research, has sponsored several scientific advisory meetings and roundtable discussions to define the issues, and it has established ongoing dialogue between the health care industry and leaders in women's health. In the process, the Society has developed a research agenda, devised strategies for increasing the ranks of women in academic medicine, and assured that understanding women's health remains a national priority.

Meanwhile, the Campaign for Women's Health (see p. 268), a coalition of diverse organizations interested in reforming the health care system to meet the needs of all women, devised a model benefits package to spell out the services women need as health care is reformed. This package, compiled by a coalition of service providers, women's health educators, physicians, and policy makers, became a working document in meetings between the Campaign and the White House Task Force on Health Care Reform. The Model Benefits Package calls for a major overhaul of the process by which health services are delivered to women. It is a comprehensive program that includes a number of measures to protect women from heart disease, among them evaluation of nutrition, exercise habits, and tobacco use; periodic medical history and physical examination; screening for heart disease risk factors; and menopause counseling.

In public policy as in research, the crusade for women's health marches forward. We feel hopeful that these trends, together with growing awareness among the medical profession and the general public, will halt the rampage of women's heart disease in its tracks.

APPENDIX

Common Medications for Treating Diseases of the Heart and Circulatory System

The following is an abbreviated guide to medications commonly prescribed to treat diseases of the heart and circulatory system, including high blood pressure and high cholesterol. For more complete information, consult the *Physicians' Desk Reference*, available in your public library, or any of the numerous drug reference guides now published for the general public. (See Some Additional Resources.)

Although we list usual dosage ranges, individual doses and the specific instructions that accompany each prescription vary widely from person to person. Cost also varies substantially depending on whether a brand-name or generic product is used, where the drug is purchased, and how various insurance plans affect your out-of-pocket expense. And while we list common side effects, you should be aware that some patients experience none. When side effects do assert themselves, their intensity can range from barely perceptible or mildly annoying at one extreme to intolerable or life-threatening at the other.

To keep you from worrying unnecessarily while helping you discern potentially dangerous side effects, we sometimes advise "Call your doctor *immediately* if . . ." *Immediately* means just that: at night, on the weekend, whenever the problem occurs. Under other circumstances we advise, "Call your doctor at the *earliest possible convenience* if. . ." Translation: Should one of these problems develop at night or on the weekend, you can safely wait to report it until the start of the next business day. All other side effects should be reported to your doctor during your next office visit.

Since contraindications, precautions, and drug interactions are many and varied, we could not list them all. However, the drugs you take can have a profound effect upon one another. It is imperative that your doctor knows about all prescription and over-the-counter drugs you use even occasionally. To protect against one of your medication's inadvertently intensifying or inhibiting the effect of another, we urge you to routinely put all the medicines in your medicine cabinet into a bag and take it with you to the doctor. This way, you won't have to worry about forgetting to mention the cough syrup you take on the rare occasion a cold keeps you up at night.

ACE INHIBITORS

	DOSE RANGE (MILLIGRAMS PER DAY)
Altace (ramipril)	1.25 to 20
Capoten (captopril)	25 to 200
Lotensin (benazepril)	5 to 80
Prinivil/Zestril (lisinopril)	5 to 30
Vasotec (enalapril maleate)	2.5 to 30
Monopril (fosinopril)	10 to 80

ACE inhibitors are prescribed to treat high blood pressure and heart failure. They prevent constriction of blood vessels and the retention of sodium and fluid. Take ACE inhibitors on an empty stomach. Do not take this drug if you are pregnant or nursing. Side effects include cough, skin rash, loss of taste, weakness, swelling of the feet or abdomen, palpitations, and headaches. If you tend to perspire heavily, ACE inhibitors can cause excessively low blood pressure.

ALPHA BLOCKERS

	DOSE RANGE (MILLIGRAMS PER DAY)
Cardura (doxazosin)	1 to 16
Hytrin (terazosin hydrochloride)	1 to 5
Minipress (prazosin hydrochloride)	1 to 15

Alpha adrenergic blockers lower high blood pressure by dilating the blood vessels. These drugs are not recommended if you are pregnant or nursing. Side effects include fainting, dizziness, headache, palpitations, fatigue, nausea, weakness, and drowsiness. Call your doctor immediately if you faint.

ANTICOAGULANTS

Coumadin/Panwarfarin (warfarin sodium)	2 to 10 milligrams per day

Warfarin prevents blood clot formation. It takes thirty-six to seventy-two hours after the initial dose to work. Do not take warfarin if you have high blood pressure, liver or kidney disease, or polycythemia. Use this drug only under strict medical supervision if you are pregnant, nursing, or have congestive heart failure. Ask your doctor how to manage cuts and other injuries. Consult your doctor about drinking alcoholic beverages and eating leafy green vegetables and other foods high in vitamin K. Maintain your dosage schedule meticulously. Unless your doctor tells you otherwise, avoid aspirin, penicillin, and phenylbutazone (Butazolidin). Side effects include excessive bleeding or a tendency to bruise easily; headaches; paralysis; chest, joint, or abdominal pain; shortness of breath; difficulty breathing or swallowing; or unexplained swelling. Call your doctor immediately if you experience unusual or uncontrollable bleeding, paralysis, headaches, joint or abdominal pain, or significant difficulty breathing.

ANTIHYPERTENSIVES

	DOSE RANGE (MILLIGRAMS PER DAY)
Aldomet (methyldopa)	250 to 1500
Catapres (clonidine)	0.1 to 1.0
Hylorel (guanadrel sulfate)	10 to 100
Tenex (guanfacine hydrochloride)	1 to 3
Wytensin (guanabenz acetate)	4 to 32

These drugs lower high blood pressure by dilating the blood vessels. Do not take Aldomet if you are allergic to sulfa or have liver disease. Do not discontinue these drugs suddenly. If you are pregnant or nursing, use these drugs only under strict medical supervision. Ask your doctor about the advisability of drinking alcoholic beverages. Consult your doctor before taking antidepressants; over-the-counter cold, allergy, or asthma medications; or any other heart or blood pressure medication. Side effects include drowsiness, depression, sexual dysfunction, fatigue, dizziness, dry mouth, stuffy nose, fever, upset stomach, change in bowel habits (some drugs cause constipation, others cause diarrhea), rash, weight gain, and fluid retention.

ANTIARRHYTHMICS

	DOSE RANGE (MILLIGRAMS PER DAY)
Cardioquin/Quinaglute/Quinidex (quinidine)	600 to 4,000
Mexitil (mexiletine hydrochloride)	400 to 1,200
Norpace (disopyramide phosphate)	400 to 800
Procan/Pronestyl (procainamide hydrochloride)	1,500 to 6,000
Rythmol (propafenone hydrochloride)	450 to 900
Tambocor (flecainide acetate)	100 to 400
Tonocard (tocainide hydrochloride)	1,200 to 2,400

Antiarrhythmics treat irregular heart rhythms by altering the conduction patterns in the heart. These drugs are not recommended if you are pregnant or nursing. If you have kidney or liver disease, use these drugs only under strict supervision of your physician. Take quinidine drugs, procainamides, and disopyramide on an empty stomach. Take all others with food or milk to reduce stomach irritation. Be sure your physician knows if you are a vegetarian or consume a lot of milk and/or vegetables. Take antacids only with your doctor's permission. Side effects include dizziness, nausea, vomiting, change in bowel habits (some drugs cause constipation, others cause diarrhea), fatigue, blurred vision, headache, congestive heart failure, indigestion, palpitations, insomnia, tremor, and rash. Call your doctor *immediately* if you experience dizziness or the symptoms of congestive heart failure (swollen ankles, unusual fatigue or shortness of breath, coughing up blood). Call your doctor at the *earliest possible convenience* if you develop a rash or insomnia.

BETA BLOCKERS

	DOSE RANGE (MILLIGRAMS PER DAY)
Blocadren (timolol maleate)	10 to 60
Corgard (nadolol)	40 to 240
Inderal (propranolol hydrochloride)	40 to 320
Kerlone (betaxolol hydrochloride)	10 to 20
Levatol (penbutolol sulfate)	20 to 80
Lopressor (metoprolol tartrate)	100 to 400
Sectral (acebutolol hydrochloride)	200 to 1,200
Tenormin (atenolol)	25 to 150
Visken (pindolol)	10 to 40

Beta blockers are prescribed to treat angina, arrhythmias, and/or high blood pressure. Do not take these drugs if you are pregnant or nursing. These drugs can prolong the effects of insulin in diabetics and diminish the ability of bronchodilators to relieve asthma. Side effects include insomnia, nightmares, nausea, fatigue, slow pulse, weakness, asthmatic attacks, cold hands and feet, dizziness, sexual dysfunction, and elevated cholesterol and blood sugar levels. Call your doctor *immediately* if you develop asthma or become dizzy. Call your doctor at the *earliest possible convenience* if you experience nightmares or sexual dysfunction.

CALCIUM CHANNEL BLOCKERS

	DOSE RANGE (MILLIGRAMS PER DAY)
Adalat/Procardia (nifedipine)	30 to 120
Cardizem (diltiazem hydrochloride)	60 to 360
Cardene (nicardipine hydrochloride)	60 to 120
Calan/Isoptin, Verelan (verapamil hydrochloride)	120 to 480
DynaCirc (isradipine)	5 to 20
Vascor (bepridil)	200 to 400
Plendil (felodipine)	5 to 20

Calcium channel blockers are used to treat angina, high blood pressure, and some arrhythmias. The preparations dilate the coronary arteries and lower blood pressure by inhibiting the passage of calcium into the heart and muscle cells. In the process, some irregular heart rhythms are also suppressed. Do not take these drugs if you are pregnant or nursing, if your heart rate is slow, or if you have advanced heart block or congestive heart failure. Take calcium channel blockers with milk or food to decrease stomach irritation. A high-fat diet may decrease the effectiveness of nicardipine (Cardene). Ask your doctor about drinking alcoholic beverages. Side effects include fluid retention, dizziness, palpitations, headache, flushes, and rash. Diltiazem and verapamil may also cause constipation. Call your doctor immediately if you experience dizziness. Call your doctor at the earliest possible convenience if you develop a rash.

DIGITALIS COMPOUNDS

	DOSE RANGE (MILLIGRAMS PER DAY)
Crystodigin (digitoxin)	0.05 to .30
Lanoxin/Lanoxicaps (digoxin)	0.05 to .35

Digitalis relieves congestive heart failure by strengthening the heart's pumping force and thereby increasing the outflow of blood. It also corrects fast, irregular heart action by decreasing electrical conduction. If you are pregnant or nursing, use these drugs only under strict medical supervision. If you take these drugs, you must be monitored closely by your physician because they can build up in the blood to toxic levels. Take antacids and over-the-counter cold remedies only with the advice of your physician. If you take Lanoxin, a high-fiber diet might reduce the drug's effectiveness. Side effects include fatigue, weakness, headache, irregular heart rhythms, unusually slow heart rate, nausea, vomiting, and loss of appetite. Call your doctor immediately if your heart rate becomes unusually slow.

DIURETICS

	DOSE RANGE (MILLIGRAMS PER DAY)
Thiazide Diuretics	
Diuril (chlorothiazide)	500 to 2,000
Esidrix/HydroDIURIL (hydrochlorothiazide)	12.5 to 50
Hygroton (chlorthalidone)	25 to 100
Lozol (indapamide)	2.5 to 5.0
Zaroxolyn (metolazone)	0.5 to 5.0
Potassium-sparing Diuretics	
Aldactone (spironolactone)	50 to 100
Dyrenium (triamterene)	200 to 300
Midamor (amiloride hydrochloride)	5 to 20
Loop Diuretics	
Bumex (bumetanide)	0.5 to 5.0
Edecrin (ethacrynic acid)	50 to 100
Lasix (furosemide)	20 to 80

Diuretics control high blood pressure and fluid retention by increasing the excretion of sodium and water. If you take diuretics, do not drink alcohol without the express permission of your physician. Since different diuretics affect the body's ability to retain potassium in different ways, consult your physician about consuming potassium-rich foods, also about using salt substitutes, which can affect calcium levels. Take these drugs with food or milk to decrease stomach irritation. Do not take any of these drugs if you are nursing. Do not take Aldactone, Dyrenium, or Midamor if you are pregnant or suffer from menstrual abnormalities or breast engorgement. If you are pregnant, take other diuretics only under strict medical supervision. Side effects of diuretics include drowsiness, dizziness, light-headedness, dehydration, electrolyte imbalances, gout, nausea, vomiting, cramping, joint pain, hearing loss, sexual dysfunction, blood sugar abnormalities, and elevated cholesterol and lipoprotein levels. Call your doctor *immediately* if you become dizzy or light-headed, if you vomit, or if you suffer a loss of hearing. Call your doctor at the *earliest possible convenience* if you develop muscle cramps.

HEMORRHEOLOGIC AGENTS

Trental (pentoxifylline)	800 to 1,200 milligrams per day

Trental improves blood flow to the extremities by reducing the viscosity of the blood. Do not take this drug if you cannot tolerate caffeine. Do not take this drug if you are pregnant or nursing. Side effects include chest pain, nausea, indigestion, vomiting, dizziness, and headaches. If you have coronary artery disease, the drug may cause angina, low blood pressure, or irregular heartbeat.

LIPID-LOWERING DRUGS

	DOSE RANGE
Colestid (colestipol hydrochloride)	5 to 30 grams per day
Lopid (gemfibrozil)	600 to 1,200 milligrams per day
Lorelco (probucol)	1,000 milligrams per day in divided doses
Mevacor (lovastatin)	20 to 80 milligrams per day
Nia-Bid/Niacor/Nicobid (niacin)	1 to 3 grams per day
Pravachol (pravastatin)	10 to 40 milligrams per day
Questran (cholestyramine)	9 to 54 grams per day
Questran Light (cholestyramine)	5 to 30 grams per day
Zocor (simvastatin)	10 to 40 milligrams per day

These drugs lower cholesterol, low-density lipoproteins, and/or triglyceride levels, depending on the drug. They interfere with the metabolism of blood fats in various ways. Do not take these drugs if you have severe liver or kidney disease, if you are pregnant, or if you are nursing.

Colestid and Questran can aggravate constipation and prevent absorption of other medications. Talk to your doctor about scheduling your dosages to assure the full benefit of each drug you take.

Take Lopid thirty minutes before breakfast and/or dinner.

Take Lorelco with food or milk to increase the drug's absorption. Make sure your doctor knows if you take antidepressants.

Take Mevacor with your evening meal. Early concerns about serious side effects from this drug, especially liver disease and cataracts, appear unfounded. This drug can be troublesome if you suffer from alcoholism, low blood pressure, acute infection, visual disturbances, uncontrolled seizures, or if you experience trauma or major surgery.

Niacin can be troublesome if you have ulcers, gout, liver disease, glaucoma, or diabetes, and it can cause hepatitis. Although niacin can be purchased over the counter, it has some potentially serious interactions with other drugs. Take niacin only under strict medical supervision.

Side effects of all lipid-lowering agents include nausea, vomiting, diarrhea, constipation, flatulence, and abdominal discomfort.

NITRATES

	DOSE RANGE (MILLIGRAMS PER DAY)
Cardilate (erythrityl tetranitrate)	15 to 100
Iso-Bid/Isordil/Sorbitrate (isosorbide dinitrate)	10 to 160
Nitro-Bid/Nitrospan/Nitrostat Transderm (nitroglycerin)	10 to 40
Peritrate (pentaerythritol tetranitrate)	40 to 160

Nitrates prevent and relieve angina by dilating the coronary arteries. They also ease congestive heart failure by increasing blood flow out of the heart. Do not take these drugs if you suffer from severe anemia. If you are pregnant or nursing or if you suffer from glaucoma, use nitrates only under strict supervision of your physician. Do not take nitrates with food. Do not discontinue these drugs rapidly. If you use a nitroglycerin patch, you must take your patch off for several hours each day so that your body continues to absorb the drug effectively without building up a tolerance to it. Ask your physician how many hours each day you should go without your patch. Consult your physician about the advisability of drinking alcoholic beverages. Side effects include headache, dizziness, low blood pressure, and rapid heartbeat. Call your doctor at the *earliest possible convenience* if you experience the symptoms of low blood pressure (light-headedness during exercise or upon rising from bed or chair) or if your heart rate becomes unusually rapid.

PLATELET INHIBITORS

	DOSE RANGE (MILLIGRAMS PER DAY)
aspirin	175 to 325
Persantine (dipyridamole)	100 to 400

Aspirin is prescribed to prevent heart attacks. Aspirin and Persantine, which prevent platelets from clumping together, are prescribed to prevent strokes and to discourage blood clot formation following heart attacks, heart surgery, and angioplasty. If you are pregnant or if you have low blood pressure or a problem with your blood platelets, use these drugs only under close medical supervision. Do not drink alcoholic beverages or take ibuprofen (Advil or Nuprin) without consulting your physician. Take aspirin with food to prevent stomach irritation. Do not take Persantine with food. Side effects of aspirin include stomach irritation and bleeding. Side effects of Persantine include headache, dizziness, nausea, low blood pressure, and stomach irritation.

VASODILATORS

	DOSE RANGE (MILLIGRAMS PER DAY)
Apresoline (hydralazine hydrochloride)	40 to 400
Loniten (minoxidil)	10 to 40

Vasodilators, used in combination with a diuretic, treat high blood pressure by dilating the peripheral blood vessels. Do not take Apresoline if you have coronary heart disease or if you have a mitral valve defect caused by rheumatic heart disease. Do not use these drugs if you are pregnant or nursing. Do not discontinue taking these drugs abruptly. Ask your physician how much caffeine is safe for you to consume and whether you may drink alcoholic beverages. Use ibuprofen (Advil, Nuprin, etc.) and over-the-counter cold, allergy, and asthma medications only under your physician's supervision. Take Apresoline with food to increase its absorption. Side effects include rapid heartbeat, water retention, dizziness, headache, drowsiness, nausea, vomiting, and diarrhea. In addition, Loniten may cause hair growth and contribute to congestive heart failure. Call your doctor immediately if you become dizzy or experience new or unusually severe difficulty breathing. Call your doctor at the earliest possible convenience if your heart rate accelerates unusually or if your ankles become swollen.

GLOSSARY

Acute myocardial infarction: Also called a heart attack. The death of a portion of heart muscle as the result of prolonged cessation of blood flow to the area.

Aneurysm: A weakened protrusion, or bubble, that forms in the wall of a blood vessel, usually an artery. When these aneurysms rupture, the result is often fatal. Aneurysms can also occur in the heart muscle as a consequence of a heart attack. These protrusions of scarred, nonfunctional muscle trap blood in the heart and prevent efficient circulation. Aneurysms of both the blood vessels and the heart muscle can be repaired surgically.

Angina: (*See also* unstable angina.) Pain caused by temporary insufficiency of blood flow to a portion of the heart muscle. Often the pain comes with physical or emotional stress and subsides when the stress abates.

Angiography: (*See also* cardiac catheterization.) A diagnostic X-ray study of the blood vessels during which a radiopaque dye is injected into the vessels via a catheter to heighten their visibility on the film. When applied to the heart, "angiography" is commonly used synonymously with "cardiac catheterization," although, technically speaking, the latter means passing a thin tube (catheter) into the heart via a vein or artery so that any of several kinds of studies can be performed. Also called arteriography.

Angioplasty: A procedure designed to widen narrowed arteries and performed via a catheter. Balloons, lasers, various cutting devices, and stents may be utilized.

Angioscopy: Visualization of the interior of a blood vessel with a microscope fixed to the end of a flexible catheter.

Anticoagulant: A drug, such as heparin or warfarin, that impedes the clotting capability of blood. Although these drugs are commonly called "blood thinners," this term is technically inaccurate.

Aorta: The largest artery in the body. This vessel carries oxygen-rich blood from the heart upward toward the head and downward into the trunk to be distributed throughout the body.

Aortic valve: A three-leaflet valve controlling the exit of oxygen-rich blood from the lower left chamber of the heart into the aorta.

Arrhythmia: Disturbance in the rhythm of the heartbeat.

Arteriogram: See angiogram *and* cardiac catheterization.

Arteriosclerosis: See atherosclerosis.

Artery: A blood vessel carrying oxygen-rich blood away from the heart.

Asymptomatic: Without symptoms.

Atherectomy: Removal of the fatty deposits and other obstructions on the inside of an artery via a catheter.

Atherosclerosis: Hardening and thickening of the artery walls caused by accumulation of blood fats, fibrous tissue, and calcium deposits. Sometimes called arteriosclerosis, although, technically speaking, atherosclerosis is one form of arteriosclerosis.

Atrial septal defect: A hole in the wall (septum) separating the two upper chambers of the heart.

Atrium: One of two upper chambers of the heart. The left atrium receives oxygen-rich blood from the lungs. The right atrium receives waste-laden blood from the central veins of the body.

Autoimmune response: The process by which the immune system attacks the body's own tissues.

Blood pressure: The force of blood beating against the artery walls.

Bradycardia: An abnormally slow heartbeat.

Bruit: (Pronounced BRU-ee.) The sound of turbulent blood flow (*see* turbulence) as detected by stethoscope.

Bypass: See coronary artery bypass.

Cardiac catheterization: (*See also* angiography.) Passage of a catheter into the heart through an arm or groin vessel in order to detect abnormalities in the coronary arteries and chambers of the heart, determine blood pressures within the heart, and obtain blood samples.

Cardiovascular: Pertaining to the heart and blood vessels.

Carotid arteries: The main vessels carrying oxygen-rich blood into the head.

Catheter: A thin, flexible tube inserted into a blood vessel and used in various procedures, including angiography, angioplasty, and atherectomy.

Cholesterol (See also lipoprotein.) A fatlike substance made by the human body and ingested with animal food products. The body utilizes cholesterol in building and repairing its tissues. Excess cholesterol forms fatty deposits in the arteries.

Claudication: Pain in the hip, thigh, or calf muscles that occurs while walking but subsides with rest. It is caused by a blockage or stiffening of the arteries that feed the legs, which prevents adequate blood flow.

Collateral circulation: Natural bypasses the body creates to keep blood flowing around blockages in the coronary arteries.

Congestive heart failure: Loss of pumping power as a result of cumulative damage to the heart.

Coronary arteries: The blood vessels that feed the heart muscle.

Coronary artery bypass: A surgical procedure that permits blood to circumvent an obstruction in the coronary arteries by traveling directly from the aorta to a branch of the coronary artery beyond the obstruction.

CPR, or cardiopulmonary resuscitation: A lifesaving first-aid technique used when the heart stops beating. It involves mouth-to-mouth breathing, which supplies oxygen to the lungs, and rhythmic application of pressure to the chest, which keeps blood circulating.

Defibrillation: The process of restoring a quivering, inefficient heartbeat to normal rhythm.

Denial: The psychological process by which people consciously or unconsciously filter out information that is threatening.

Depression: A psychological state often characterized by some combination of the following: dejected mood, lack of interest in normally stimulating activities, sleep and appetite disturbances, low energy, difficulties thinking and concentrating, and feelings of inadequacy and guilt.

Diastolic: Pertaining to the relaxation phase of the heartbeat.

Distal: Farthest from the center, from the midline, or from the trunk. For example, the foot is distal to the hip.

Doppler: See ultrasound.

Dyspnea: (Pronounced DIS-nee-uh.) Shortness of breath.

Echocardiogram: See ultrasound.

Edema: Abnormal retention of fluid in the body tissues. When fluid collects in the ankles and abdomen, it becomes apparent as swelling. When fluid collects in the lungs, breathing becomes difficult.

Electrocardiogram, or EKG: A tracing of the electrical activity of the heart.

Electrophysiology study: A procedure similar to cardiac catheterization in which EKG leads are threaded through the blood vessels to capture electrical tracings from areas of the heart that external EKG leads cannot detect.

Embolism: Obstruction of a blood vessel by a foreign substance, usually a blood clot (thromboembolism).

Endarterectomy: Surgical removal of the inner layer of an artery when it has become thickened and narrowed by plaque or fatty deposits.

Endocarditis: An infection of the lining of the heart.

Endovascular: Pertaining to the inside of blood vessels.

Fibrillation: Uncontrollable quivering of the heart. Atrial fibrillation is common and often easy to treat. Ventricular fibrillation is life threatening.

Gaited exercise test: An assessment of the coronary arteries' ability to meet the heart's increasing demand for blood. During the test, blood pressure, breathing, and heart function are monitored. Also called a stress test or a stress EKG.

Heart attack: See acute myocardial infarction.

Heart block: An abnormal heart rhythm caused by failure of the electrical impulses to move from one area of the heart to another in a timely or efficient manner.

Heart failure: See congestive heart failure.

Internal mammary artery: One of two arteries that feed the chest wall. It is often used to create coronary artery bypass grafts.

Intravascular ultrasound: A technique whereby a miniature ultrasound device affixed to a catheter captures two-dimensional images from within a blood vessel.

Ischemia: Insufficient oxygen supply to a part of the body.

Laser: A device that emits a very strong, very precise beam of light, sometimes used as a surgical tool.

Lesion: An area of diseased tissue; a wound.

Lipid: Fats (e.g., triglycerides) or fatlike (e.g., cholesterol) substances.

Lipoprotein: A protein molecule that serves as a transportation vehicle for blood lipids. Low-density lipoproteins carry cholesterol from the liver into the bloodstream. High-density lipoproteins remove cholesterol from the bloodstream and return them to the liver.

Lumen: The channel inside an artery or vein.

Mitral valve: The two-leaflet valve that controls blood flow between the upper and lower chambers on the left side of the heart.

Mitral valve prolapse: A condition, rarely serious, caused by the protrusion of the mitral valve leaflets into the left atrium above when the valve opens in response to the contraction of the left ventricle.

Murmur: The sound of blood moving inefficiently through the valves of the heart.

Myocardial infarction: See acute myocardial infarction.

Occlusion: The closure of a passage. For example, the obstruction of a blood vessel by plaque, spasm, or blood clot.

Pacemaker: An electrical device used to maintain the heartbeat at a desired rate when the heart cannot do so independently.

Percutaneous: Performed through the skin.

Plaque: A buildup of debris in a blood vessel.

Prinzmetal's angina: See variant angina.

Proximal: Nearest the point of attachment or center of the body. For example, the shoulder is proximal to the hand.

Pulmonary: Pertaining to the lungs.

Rales: The crackling sound heard through the stethoscope when fluid is present in the tissues of the lung.

Regurgitation: The back flow of blood through a valve that does not close completely.

Renal: Pertaining to the kidneys.

Restenosis: The recurrence of a narrowing or constriction of a passage.

Rheumatic heart disease: The long-term complication of untreated streptococcal infection such as strep throat. It can culminate in valve damage requiring open-heart surgery.

Saphenous vein: The longest vein in the body, extending from the foot to the groin. This vein is commonly used for coronary artery bypass grafts.

Septum: The vertical structure separating the right chambers of the heart from the left.

Silent heart disease: The development of coronary artery blockages and/or the occurrence of a heart attack without the telltale pain.

Stenosis: Constriction or narrowing of a blood vessel, a heart valve, or other passage.

Stent: A wire mesh support fitted inside an artery to keep the artery open.

Stress test: See gaited exercise test.

Stroke: Injury to the brain caused by insufficient blood flow through the carotid arteries or by a hemorrhage of a blood vessel in the brain.

Syncope: Dizziness or fainting as a result of insufficient blood flow to the brain.

Syndrome X: A painful but benign heart condition caused by the inability of some of the heart's capillaries to dilate normally.

Systolic: Pertaining to the contraction phase of the heartbeat.

Tachycardia: An abnormally rapid heartbeat.

Thallium stress test: A test done to identify areas of heart muscle that receive diminished blood supply, during physical exertion. Thallium, a metallic element, is injected along with a vessel dilator. A gaited exercise EKG is performed and a scan is taken to view the distribution of blood through the heart muscle.

Thromboembolism: The blocking of a blood vessel by a blood clot that has broken loose from its site of formation.

Thrombosis: Formation, development, or existence of a blood clot within a blood vessel.

Transducer: A device that converts one form of energy to another. It is used in medical electronics to receive energy from sound or pressure and relay it as an electrical impulse to a recording device.

Triglycerides: A kind of blood fat implicated in the development of coronary heart disease.

Turbulence: Inefficient blood flow caused by plaque in the arteries, which churns up the blood; or back flow through improperly closing valves.

Ultrasound: The utilization of sound wave technology to image the body. An ultrasound examination of the heart is called an echocardiogram. Doppler technology, incorporated into an ultrasound study, portrays blood flow by interpreting the changing length of sound waves reflected by the moving blood.

Unstable angina: An advanced state of angina characterized by pain that occurs at rest as well as with activity.

Variant angina: Also called Prinzmetal's angina. Pain that occurs when a coronary artery goes into spasm, preventing blood flow to a portion of the heart muscle.

Vein: A blood vessel carrying waste-laden blood toward the heart.

Ventricle: One of two lower heart chambers. The left ventricle, the largest and most important chamber of the heart, sends oxygen-rich blood out into the body. The right ventricle sends waste-laden blood to the lungs for cleansing.

SOME ADDITIONAL RESOURCES

Bensen, Herbert, M.D., and Miriam Z. Klipper. *The Relaxation Response* (New York: Avon Books, 1976). A classic in the theory and practice of one type of meditation.

Brody, Jane. *Good Food Gourmet* (New York: W. W. Norton, 1990). The latest in Jane Brody's Good Food series, this collection features five hundred interesting recipes relatively low in fat.

Cohan, Carol, June B. Pimm, and James R. Jude. *A Patient's Guide to Heart Surgery* (New York: HarperCollins, 1991). A detailed exploration of the medical, practical, and emotional aspects of heart surgery from the time surgery is recommended until late in the recuperation process.

Delaney, Sue. *Women Smokers Can Quit: A Different Approach* (Evanston, Ill.: Women's Healthcare Press, 1989). A former smoker tackles particularly female problems associated with kicking the habit, such as fear of gaining weight.

Farquhar, John W., and Gene A. Spiller. *The Last Puff* (New York: W. W. Norton, 1990). Thirty personal success stories from former smokers.

Greenberg, Jerrold S. *Managing Stress: A Personal Guide* (Dubuque, Iowa: Wm. C. Brown Publishers, 1984). A comprehensive overview of stress management techniques with instruction in meditation, self-hypnosis, progressive relaxation, and more.

Grundy, Scott M., M.D., Ph.D., and Mary Winston, Ed.D., R.D., eds. *The American Heart Association Low-Fat, Low-Cholesterol Cookbook* (New York: Times Books, 1989). An accessible introduction to low-fat cooking, this volume is filled with healthful adaptations of favorite American recipes. Wait till you see the desserts!

Harvard Heart Letter. Thomas H. Lee, M.D., and Lee Goldman, M.D., co-editors., and *Harvard Health Letter*, William Ira Bennett, M.D., ed. (Boston, Mass.: Harvard Medical School Health Publications Group). In a market brimming with monthly health newsletters, these two are among the best.

Horowitz, Lawrence C., M.D. *Taking Charge of Your Medical Fate.* (New York: Random House, 1988). A discussion of why it is important to take an active role in your medical care and guidance for accomplishing the task.

Long, James W., M.D. *The Essential Guide to Prescriptions* (New York: Harper-Collins 1991). Comprehensive drug information written specifically for the general public and updated annually.

Milas, Judy, M.S., R.D. *Here's to Your Heart: The Arizona Heart Institute and Foundation's Cookbook Plus* (Phoenix: Arizona Heart Institute and Foundation, 1992). Nutritional information for adults and children; sections on diabetes, weight control, exercise, and more. For ordering information, call 800-345-4278.

Natow, Annette, Ph.D., R.D., and Jo-Ann Heslin, M.A., R.D. *The Fat Counter* (New York: Pocket Books, 1989). Fat and calorie values for over ten thousand foods.

Ornish, Dr. Dean. *Dr. Dean Ornish's Program for Reversing Heart Disease* (New York: Random House, 1990). How to use diet, exercise, and stress reduction to reverse heart disease. Also a wealth of interesting, innovative, very low fat recipes.

Piscatella, Joseph. *Controlling Your Fat Tooth* (New York: Workman Press, 1991); *Choices for a Healthy Heart* (New York: Workman Press, 1987). Both volumes contain over two hundred easy, low-fat recipes. But perhaps their greatest value is in the life-style information they provide.

Shofer, Lois M., Ph.D. *The American College of Sports Medicine Fitness Book* (Champaign, Ill.: Human Kinetics Publishers, 1992). A beginner's guide to healthy exercise and a reference for health and fitness professionals. Includes a test to assess your fitness level and step-by-step instructions for creating and following a program that's appropriate for you.

Smart Heart, an animated video for children about cholesterol, fats, exercise, and smoking. Also *Heart Healthy Lessons for Children,* a health and nutrition education program, including visual aids and activities, designed for easy integration into grade school curricula. Both produced by Arizona Heart Institute. For ordering information call Judy Milas at 800-345-4278.

Sunshine, Linda, and John W. Wright. *The Best Hospitals in America* (New York: Henry Holt and Co., 1987). A discussion of what constitutes an outstanding hospital and an annotated listing of sixty-four superb institutions.

Tannen, Deborah. *You Just Don't Understand: Women and Men in Conversation* (New York: William Morrow and Company, 1990). This analysis of men's and women's different styles of communication promotes better understanding of and communication between the sexes and may help you communicate more effectively with medical personnel and your family.

Tufts University Diet and Nutrition Letter. Stanley N. Gershoff, Ph.D., ed. (Medford, Mass.: Tufts University School of Nutrition). A monthly newsletter promulgating the most recent nutrition research.

Williams, Redford, M.D. *The Trusting Heart* (New York: Times Books, 1989). An exploration of hostility and anger, the most pernicious facets of the Type A behavior pattern, and how to cultivate a healthier, more trusting attitude.

Index

About the Authors

EDWARD B. DIETHRICH, M.D., is director and chief of cardiovascular surgery at the Arizona Heart Institute, and is also director and chief of cardiovascular surgery and heart and lung transplantation at Humana Hospital in Phoenix, Arizona. CAROL COHAN is a medical writer whose previous work includes *A Patient's Guide to Heart Surgery: Understanding the Practical and Emotional Aspects of Heart Surgery.*